How To **GO FURTHER**

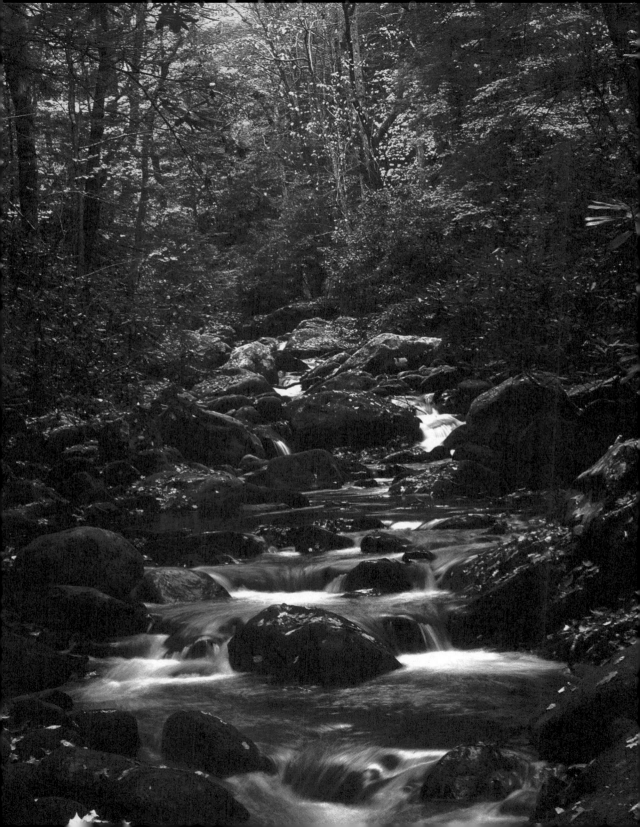

How To

GO FURTHER

A Guide to Simple Organic Living

With Woody Harrelson & Friends

Compiled & Edited by Frank Condron

HOW TO GO FURTHER

We acknowledge the financial support of the Government
of Canada through the Book Publishing Industry
Development Program for our publishing activities.

ISBN: 1-894622-39-1

Published by Warwick Publishing Inc.
161 Frederick Street, Toronto, Ontario M5A 4P3 Canada
www.warwickgp.com

Distributed in Canada by
Canadian Book Network
c/o Georgetown Terminal Warehouses
34 Armstrong Avenue
Georgetown, Ontario L7G 4R9
www.canadianbooknetwork.com

Distributed in the United States by
CDS
193 Edwards Drive
Jackson TN 38301
www.cdsbooks.com

Editor: Frank Condron
Managing Editor: Melinda Tate
Design: Clint Rogerson
Photo credits/Copyrights: See page 245

Printed and bound in Canada

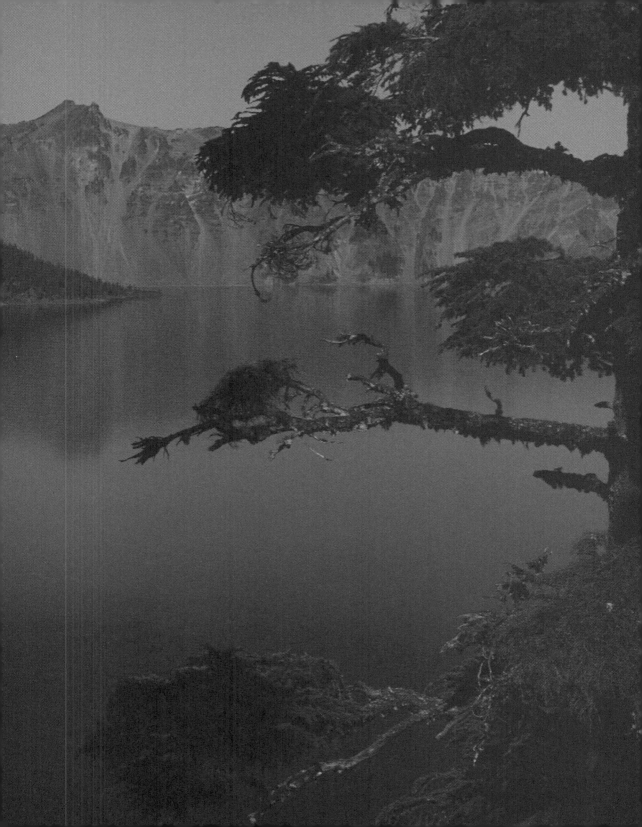

PUBLISHER'S NOTE

In making the feature documentary GO FURTHER, producer/director Ron Mann, with a small crew, followed Woody Harrelson and the SOL Tour down the West Coast from Seattle to the outskirts of Los Angeles, filming the entire journey as well as all of the appearances and impromptu speaking engagements that were made along the way. The result was more than 600 hours of footage to mine for what became a truly original and extraordinary film.

In addition, the transcripts of those 600 hours proved to be an invaluable written record of the tour and of the principles and beliefs of those who participated. Those words form the basis of this book. Writer/editor Frank Condron pored over texts of repeated lectures and public appearances, as well as the less formal conversations engaged in by SOL participants and derived repeated content categories, themes and beliefs that he methodically and faithfully stitched together into the book you are holding. These written words were then reviewed by Woody Harrelson and several members of the SOL tour, as well as by filmmaker Ron Mann, and vetted for accuracy and, less tangibly, for the comfort of the speaker himself.

Specifically, the following components of the book came together in the following manner:

- All of Woody's material: as described above, Frank Condron drew from the dozens of hours of Woody's transcripts and stitched together his thoughts and words on each of the topics discussed. From here Woody went over all of this material in close detail—adding material where necessary, striking out material he felt was incorrect or not to his liking, and concentrating on the clarity of the message. From here, Woody's changes were made and the final materials prepared for design.

- The pieces by Joe Hickey and Steve Clark were created from extensive interviews with each. From there Frank Condron wrote their stories and then each subject reviewed and changed the pieces as needed.

- The pieces by John Schaeffer, Twilly Cannon and Paul Armentano were all submitted by their authors.

- "Chocolate of the Gods Mousse" came to us via Laura and Woody's website, voiceyourself.com, with permission from its creator, Renée Loux Underkoffler of Euphoric Organics, who suggests that "it would be excellent to send people to my last book, *Living Cuisine* (Penguin-Avery) for another few hundred recipes of deliciousness."

- Throughout the book there are sidebars and factoids. These were written by Canadian writer and vegan activist Kate Harper. She was greatly aided in this task by our in-house managing editor, Melinda Tate, who, in fact, went through all of the book's materials with an eye towards consistency and accuracy.

- The photography in this book comes from a variety of sources: Ron Mann's film *Go Further* is where the majority of the images come from— we literally light-boxed a dupe print and cut out 35mm frames as they jumped at us. From there we augmented with images from various sources as listed on the copyright page. Of special note is the image of the Vietnam War supplied by my business partner, Jim Williamson, who served in 1968.

- All of the art direction and design for this book was supplied by Clint Rogerson who is in-house here at Warwick.

- In the end, thanks to the help of Woody and many members of the SOL Tour, we believe the final result is an accurate recording of the ideas expressed on that journey, and a faithful reflection of the emotions that lie at the heart of Simple Organic Living.

Nick Pitt
Publisher

KEN K

(1935

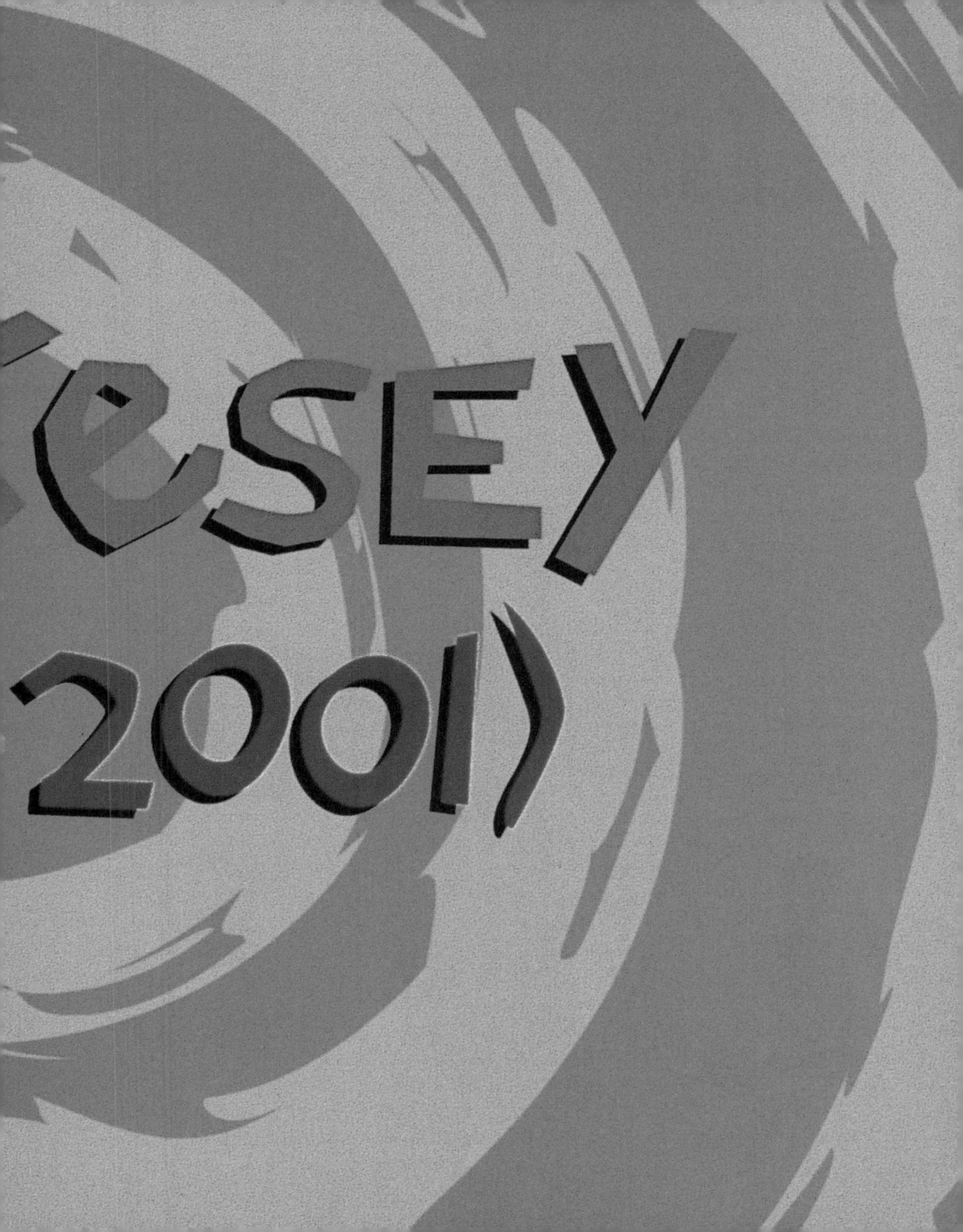
eSEY
2001

INTRODUCTION

A few years back, I experienced something that changed my life. It took place in the spring of 2001, when I embarked on a journey with some close friends that came to be known as the Simple Organic Living, or SOL, Tour.

I had no idea when it all began that our journey would have the impact it did, both on me and on the many others who were touched by its central message: to walk with a lighter footprint on the earth. But as I traveled and had the opportunity to speak to people of all ages and backgrounds, I learned there's a real desire out there to make things better, a desire for individuals to improve the quality of their personal lives, and a desire to make the world a better place to live. People are just looking for someone to hand them the right tools and show them the way.

That's essentially what we tried to do on the SOL Tour: show people how to improve their lives and sustain the planet at the same time. As time passes and more and more people hear our message, I really feel like we started something that could make a difference. The original SOL Tour ended after just thirty-four days, but I know the pursuit of a more simple organic life is a journey I'll be on for the rest of my life. I hope you'll join me.

· · ·

The whole thing actually began as just a vacation. In the spring of 2001, I was wrapping up shooting on some episodes of *Will & Grace* that I'd done and me and my brothers, Brett and Jordan, decided to take the long bike ride we'd been talking about for years. We're all into cycling, so we thought it would be cool to take off for a few weeks and just cruise some scenic highway on our bikes, stopping wherever we wanted and camping along the way.

At first we thought we'd do the Blue Ridge Parkway through North Carolina and western Tennessee. Then, on second thought, we figured it would be more convenient for everybody if we stuck to the West Coast, because that's basically where our lives were located. We finally decided to follow the coastline, about a thousand miles (1500 km) from Seattle right down to Santa Barbara. We could've gone all the way to L.A., but we all agreed we didn't want to spoil it by finishing up such a beautiful experience in the heart of Babylon.

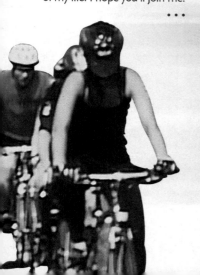

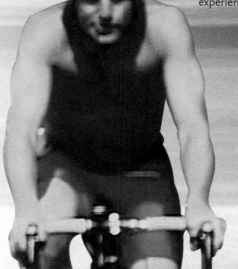

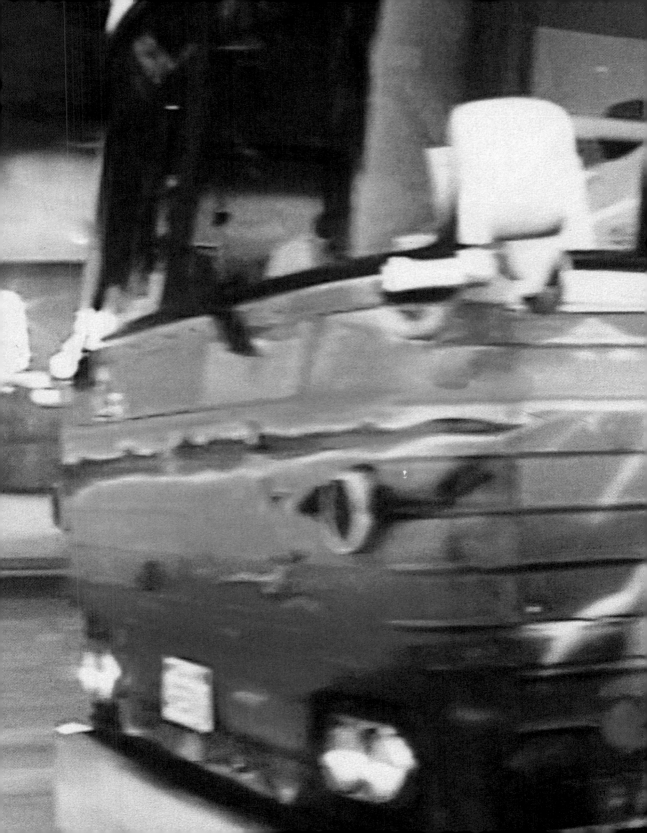

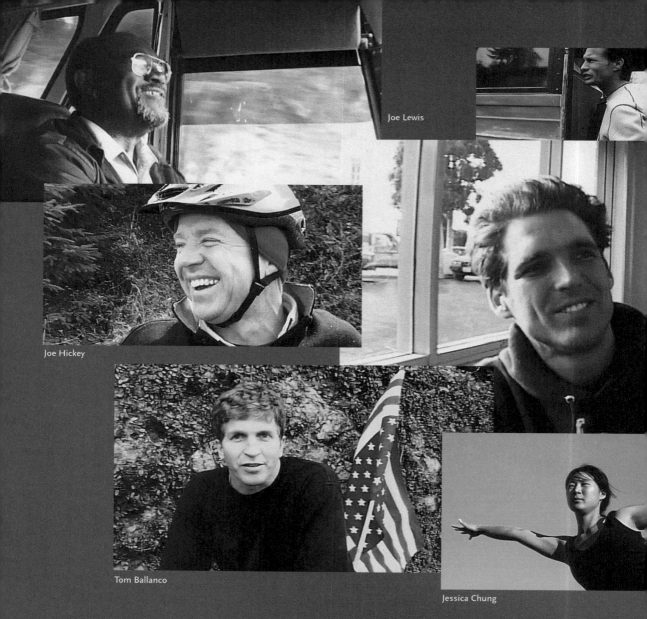

Joe Lewis

Joe Hickey

Tom Ballanco

Jessica Chung

Once we decided on the route, we began to realize this wasn't going to be just a casual bike ride. For one thing, we needed some way to carry tents and sleeping bags. Then it dawned on us that it was probably not a bad idea to bring some extra bike parts along, like tires, wheels, and chains, in case we ran into trouble in the middle of nowhere. My wife pointed out that things might get dicey if one of us crashed and we had no way to get to a hospital (advice, by the way, that turned out

to be a premonition). Then we figured, OK, maybe we should have a little van following us with all our stuff. That meant we were going to need a driver, so I recruited my old buddy Joe Lewis. I met Joe when he was my driver on *White Men Can't Jump* and he's been my regular driver on movie shoots and a dear friend ever since.

We thought we were set with Joe and the van, but then I told my environmental lawyer friend Tom Ballanco about the trip and he wanted to come. Then my friend

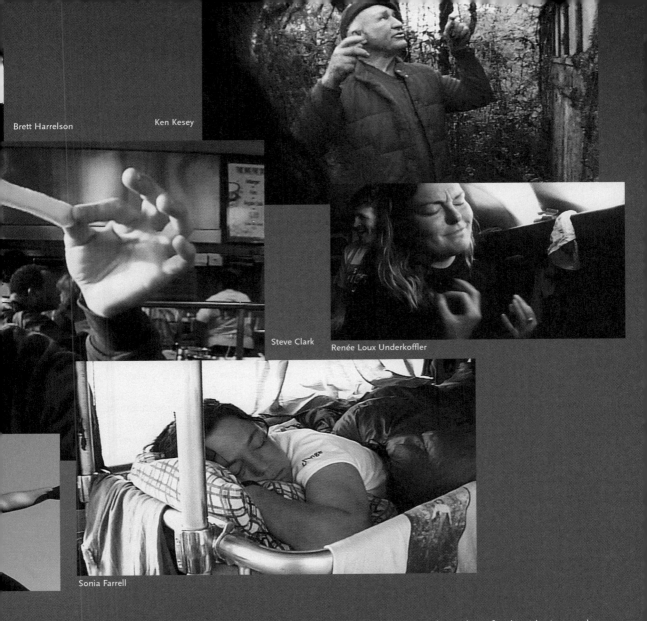

Brett Harrelson

Ken Kesey

Steve Clark

Renée Loux Underkoffler

Sonia Farrell

Joe Hickey, who I call the hub of the wheel of the hemp movement, got wind of it and he signed on. I met both Tom and Joe back in 1996, when I got into some hot water in Kentucky for planting some hemp seeds. We've been through a lot together since then, fighting the good fight for hemp and the environment, and it's like I have two more brothers with them in my life.

Actually, I probably should have known then that it wasn't going to be the quiet little bike trip we originally envisioned. With Tom and Joe along for the ride, I started to think about my experience in Kentucky and how much fun we had when we went and spoke at a local college there about the hemp movement. It wasn't anything that we really planned; we set it up that day and we each got up and just talked to the students about the dangers of corporate agriculture and the benefits of sustainable crops like hemp. The whole thing had a great energy and spontaneity to it, and there was a lot of interest in what we were doing.

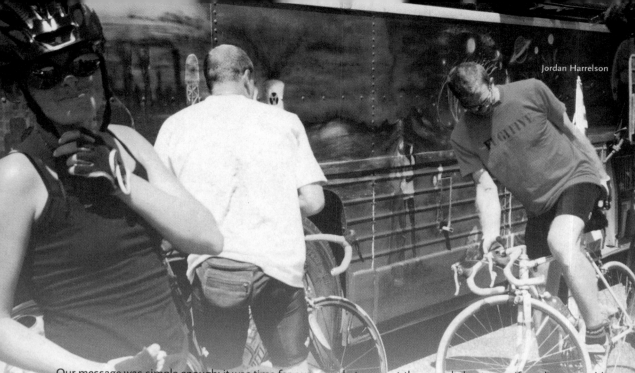

Jordan Harrelson

Our message was simple enough: it was time for our society to realize that we're in a serious situation—the planet has been trying to tell us that for years. It was clear, to us anyway, that we have to start making adjustments to the way we live if we want future generations to have any kind of future at all. Our goal, in a word, should be sustainability. The kids we spoke to really picked up on that, and I could see that there was a real hunger to hear about solutions.

The more I thought about it, the more I liked the idea of turning our bike trip into more than just a pleasure cruise. I've always had strong convictions when it comes to the hemp movement and the environment, and I've always been willing to voice those convictions. I came to the inescapable conclusion long ago that there needs to be a radical readjustment in the way we each look at ourselves and the way we look at the world. We can choose to ignore the problem, as if a coat of paint might have made the Berlin Wall easier to look at, but everyone knows that wall had to come down in the end.

That's the way I feel anyway, and the way my friends feel. But I realized unless I went out and met people and spoke to them about what I believe, I would never know just how many others felt that way. I was curious to see

what was out there, and also to see if maybe we could sow some seeds of change.

I mentioned to Tom and Joe that it might be good if we stopped off at some colleges and festivals along the way to talk about what we care about—things like diet, yoga, and living sustainably—and they were into that. So I got my assistant, Sonia, to start calling student associations to set up some dates. Word started to spread among our mutual friends about the trip, and pretty soon we added a raw food chef and a yoga instructor to our growing tribe. Before I knew what happened, the little van that was supposed to follow us had turned into a bus.

The idea of the bus really freaked me out at first. The image of a big old diesel-burning, smoke-belching coach bus following a bunch of free radicals on bikes talking about having a "lighter footprint on the earth" just didn't work for me. Then Sonia remembered reading about this guy who traveled across the country in a diesel-powered van that he retrofitted to burn cooking oil. He made it right across the country just bumming used cooking oil off McDonald's and Burger King restaurants any time he needed to fuel up. We located Josh Tickell through his book *From the Fryer to the Fuel Tank,* and he proved

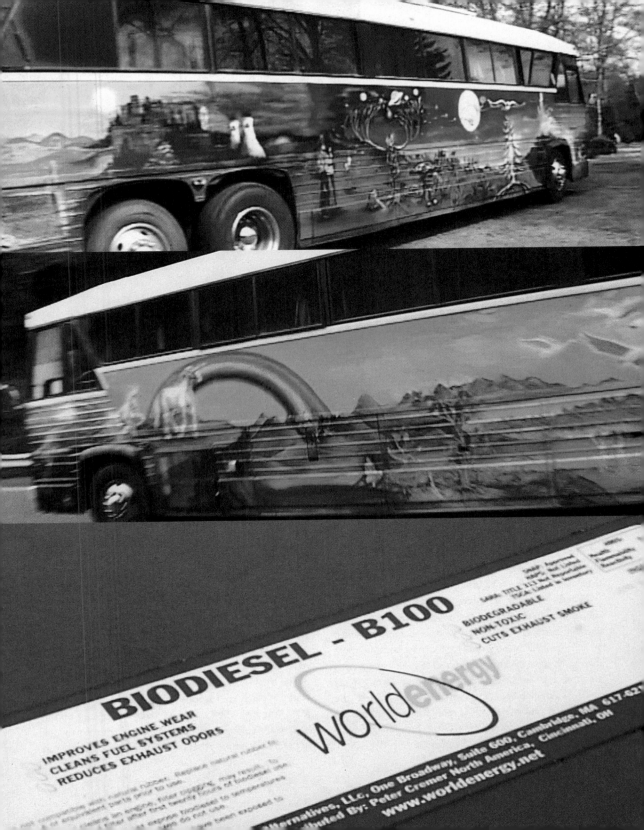

invaluable to our journey. With a little research, and some minor adjustments, we found out that our big old coach bus could run just as well on bio-fuel as it did on diesel. Better still, it could also run on vegetable oil and hemp seed oil, which fit in perfectly with our message of sustainability.

We could have been satisfied with the fact we were able to run the bus with sustainable fuel and left it at that, but we thought about it some more and decided there was a lot more we could do. So we covered the floor of the bus with sustainably harvested cork flooring and used hemp fabric to recover the walls and ceiling. Then an engineer friend of mine rigged up some solar panels on the roof that were capable of supplying electricity for all the lights, computers, cell phones, and the stereo on board. No air-conditioning though; just fresh air. Cooking, of course, wasn't a problem because everyone in the group was committed to a raw food diet, at least for the duration of the trip.

We finished it off by hand-painting a mural on the sides of the bus depicting our ultimate goal: the progression of humankind and the planet from the current state of crisis we've created to a more peaceful, sustainable future we can hand over to the new stewards—our kids. We christened our bus the Mothership, and I'm confident it is one of the most eco-conscious pieces of heavy machinery you're likely to find on the road today.

When I look back on it now, I guess if there was any one thing that made the SOL Tour come alive, it was that bus. Because of all the work we put into making it environmentally friendly, the Mothership became more than just a place to eat and sleep and store our clothes and equipment; it was the model for what we were trying to say about sustainability. And when we combined the Mothership with our traveling road show of activists on bikes, we ended up creating a living, breathing, moving example of how to walk with a lighter footprint on the earth.

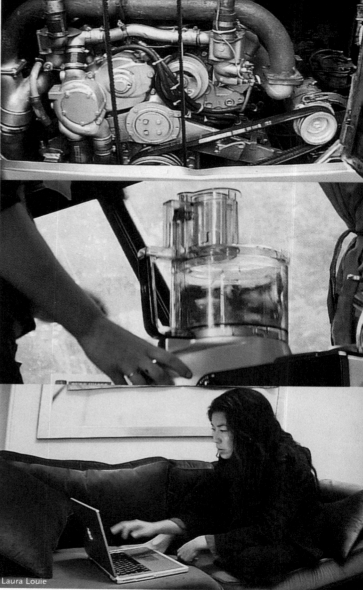

Laura Louie

It wasn't long after we started our journey—I think it was just the second or third day—when I got my first inkling of the potential of the SOL Tour. I was out on the road cycling by myself when I noticed Joe Lewis had pulled the bus into a rest stop up ahead to wait for the bikers to catch up. I stopped to chat and take a break for a few minutes when I realized cars were pulling off the highway and people were coming over to the bus to look at the mural. As the other members of our group started

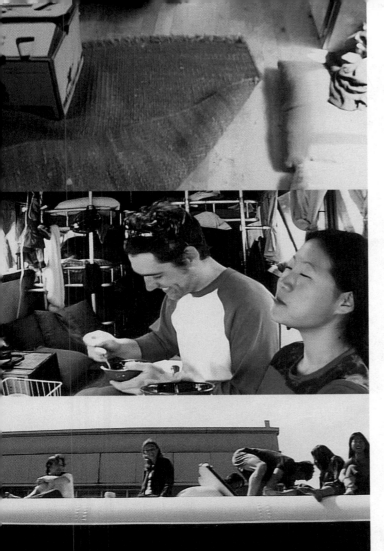

out, folks along the way actually started to look out for us, often standing by the side of the road to wave as we cycled past. Because the bus and the Tour were such perfect models for the message we were trying to send, it was really easy to get the "lighter footprint" message across whenever we stopped to talk. All we were saying was there are other ways to do things and all it takes is the will to make a change. Just like the Tour itself, sometimes the journey isn't easy and the quarters may be cramped, sometimes the ground is a little hard and the wind's a little chilly, but you can get through it all if you have the will. And the joy you experience on the other side is the trade-off.

A thousand miles is a long way to ride a bike, but I never found myself struggling to find the motivation to keep going. I fed off the fact that every day brought another opportunity to talk to someone new and plant another seed. In fact, just after we held our first lecture on the Tour, the potential of the whole thing started to sink in and a sense of responsibility began to wash over me. It wasn't negative in any way, it was just a sense of believing that what we were doing was important and that there was a reason we were called to do it, by Mother Earth or the universe or whatever. My vacation had become a mission.

The truth is, I do have a responsibility, as we all do. I know it's a lot easier to continue to do what you're doing and to reap what you're reaping. Unfortunately, I believe if we

to cycle in one after the other, people started asking us what we were doing and what the mural meant. In just a few minutes we had a little crowd of perfect strangers gathered right there by the side of the highway, and we were talking to them about how we try to live sustainably.

I was blown away by the level of curiosity and interest we encountered right from the beginning, and that level only grew as the tour progressed down the coast and the local media started to pick up on it. Once the word was continue down that path, all we're going to end up reaping is the contamination of the earth. That's why I feel we're each obligated to do as much as we, individually, can do to walk with a lighter footprint. And with that comes an additional obligation to stand up whenever we can and say, "There is another way." That's what the SOL Tour was all about, and that's why, for me at least, it'll never really come to an end.

• • •

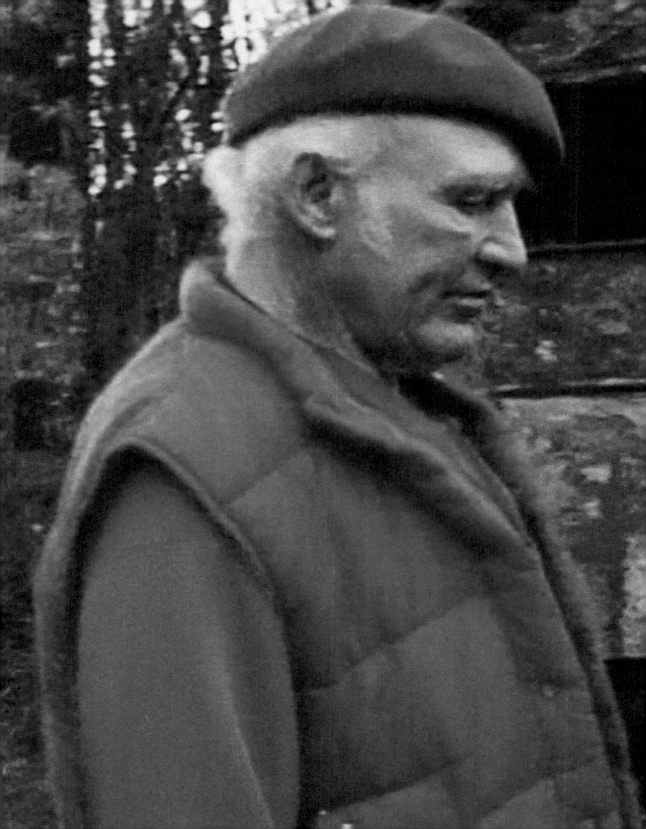

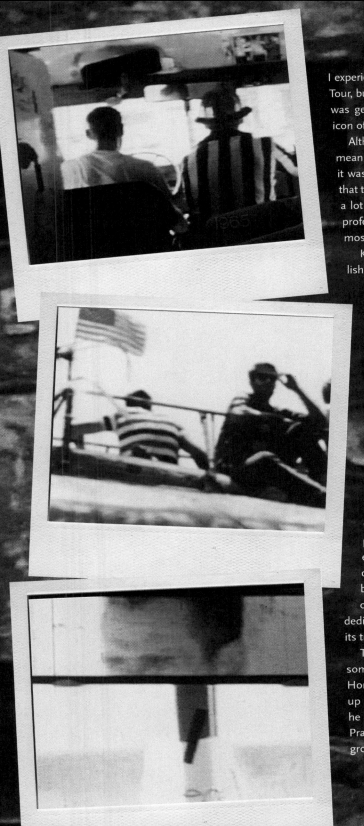

I experienced a lot of incredible moments on the SOL Tour, but without a doubt one of the most memorable was getting a chance to meet the great author and icon of the 1960s, Ken Kesey.

Although the name Ken Kesey probably doesn't mean much to most people under forty, in the 1960s it was synonymous with a lot of the social changes that took place back then. In fact, Ken Kesey can take a lot of the credit for helping to start what college professors like to call "the counterculture," and most other people know as the hippie movement.

Kesey first gained notoriety for a novel he published in 1962 called *One Flew Over The Cuckoo's Nest*. The novel was inspired by Kesey's experiences as a volunteer in a government-run research program into the effects of hallucinogenic drugs. Depending on how old you are, you might be more familiar with the movie based on it that starred Jack Nicholson. Jack played McMurphy, a bogus patient in a mental hospital who leads his fellow patients in a revolt against the oppressive Nurse Ratched.

During the research program, Kesey lived in the psychiatric wing of a VA hospital and spent his days experimenting with drugs like psilocybin mushrooms, mescaline, and LSD. The experience shocked him out of his conventional state of mind and had a profound effect on his view of America in the late 1950s. Through the prism of the "mind-expanding" drugs, he started to see dangers lurking beneath the complacency and consumerism of the time, behind the blind faith in government and the blind pursuit of personal wealth. When he left the program, he dedicated the rest of his life to shaking society out of its trance and he used his writing to make his point.

The novel was a best-seller, and Kesey used some of the money he made to buy some land in La Honda, just south of San Francisco, where he set up a commune with a group of like-minded friends he called the Merry Pranksters. Kesey and the Pranksters quickly turned the place into a breeding ground for many of the things that would become

One Flew Over the Cuckoo's Nest

Ken Kesey

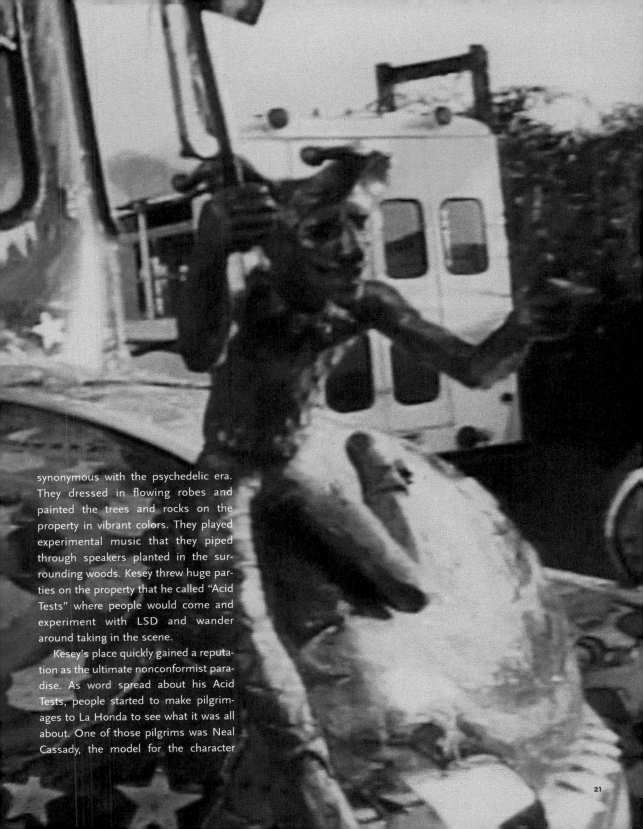

synonymous with the psychedelic era. They dressed in flowing robes and painted the trees and rocks on the property in vibrant colors. They played experimental music that they piped through speakers planted in the surrounding woods. Kesey threw huge parties on the property that he called "Acid Tests" where people would come and experiment with LSD and wander around taking in the scene.

Kesey's place quickly gained a reputation as the ultimate nonconformist paradise. As word spread about his Acid Tests, people started to make pilgrimages to La Honda to see what it was all about. One of those pilgrims was Neal Cassady, the model for the character

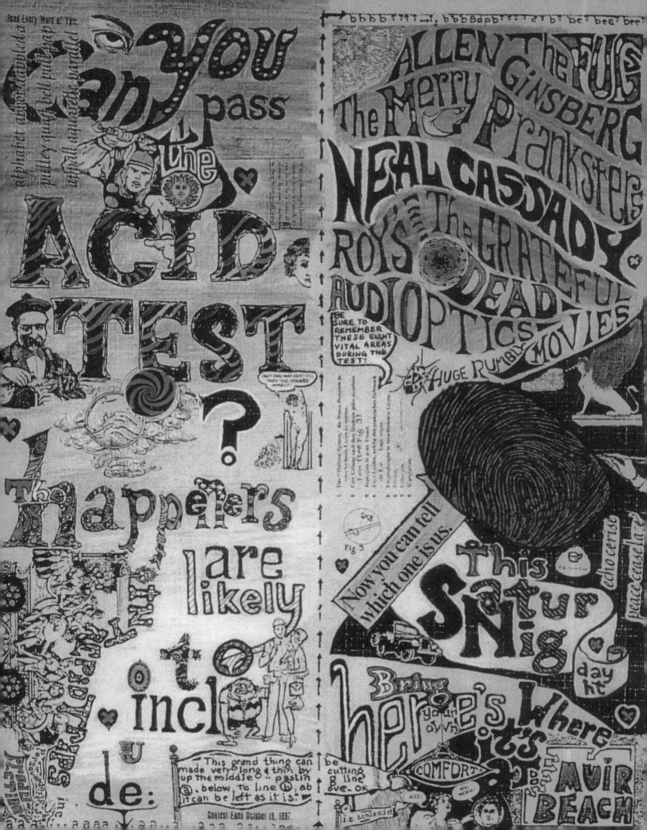

Dean Moriarty in Jack Kerouac's *On the Road*, the 1957 cult novel that set the tone for the previous generation of nonconformists, the Beats. Kesey and the Pranksters eventually started throwing Acid Tests at bigger venues around California and their ideas about art, music, fashion, and communal living started to catch on, especially in San Francisco.

In 1964, Kesey published his second novel, *Sometimes a Great Notion*. (They made a movie from that one too, about the struggles of an Oregon logging family, starring Paul Newman and Henry Fonda.) Kesey needed to travel to New York for the launch of the book, but instead of flying he bought a 1939 International Harvester school bus and turned it into a "commune on wheels" for the trip. The Pranksters took some seats out to make a sleeping area and covered the whole thing with a rainbow of Day-Glo paint, right down to the wheels. They christened their bus FURTHER, combining "future" and "farther," two words that were central to their new philosophy of living.

With Cassady at the wheel, Kesey and the Merry Pranksters set off on their journey across the country, smoking pot and dropping acid all the way. They stopped off in towns and at colleges across the Midwest to give impromptu concerts and lectures from a stage they had built on top of the bus. When confused onlookers or reporters asked Kesey what the hell the Pranksters were trying to do, he would just say they were "trying to stop the coming end of the world."

When they finally arrived in New York, Kesey and the Pranksters met with Kerouac and the poet Allen Ginsberg, two of the driving forces behind the Beat movement. With that meeting, I guess you could say the torch was symbolically passed to the next generation of nonconformists charged with saving modern society from itself. Later, Ginsberg joined Kesey and the gang for the trip up to the Castalia Institute in Millbrook, New York, to see Timothy Leary, the former Harvard psychology professor and "prophet of LSD" who had been one of the first to experiment with psychedelic drugs. With Leary's blessing, the Pranksters turned around and headed back to California.

That cross-country odyssey in 1964 was a journey of discovery for sure, probably more so for the people who saw that crazy bus than it was for Kesey and the Merry Pranksters. Actually, for probably ninety-nine per cent of the Midwestern Americans who saw the Merry Pranksters on that trip, it was likely the first time they had ever seen anyone with a beard and long hair and dressed in rainbow-colored clothes, and the first time they'd ever heard about concepts like communal living, free love, or recreational drugs. In fact, nonconformity of any kind was an alien concept to most Americans in the early 1960s. But by the time the Pranksters got back to California, they had become the crest of a wave that would sweep over the entire country over the course of the next few years. Their cause got a big boost from the writer Tom Wolfe, who rode with Kesey and the Pranksters for a while and recorded the experience in the book, *The Electric Kool-Aid Acid Test*, published in 1967, that went on to become a best-seller.

By then, the psychedelic era was in full bloom. Just as Kesey had hoped in the early 1960s, it was as though conventional society had been shaken loose and everything was changing at once. The "Summer of Love" produced music unlike anything people had ever heard before, like Jefferson Airplane's *Surrealistic Pillow* and the Beatles' *Sgt. Pepper's Lonely Hearts Club Band*, Dylan went electric, and bands like the Doors were mixing drugs and music and making hit records. The long-haired hippie look was common in big cities like San Francisco and L.A. and on college campuses, and loud colors and radical designs were the leading trend in fashion and art. In just three short years since they set out from La Honda in their rainbow-painted bus, Ken Kesey and the Merry Pranksters had become mainstream.

But more important for Kesey, by 1967 people weren't content to just follow social norms set down for them by other people. Independent thought had taken over. It was evident in the way people wore their hair and their clothes and in the music they listened to. But it was also evident in the way people were now questioning their governments and their leaders, on Vietnam, civil rights, women's rights. Regular people, especially the young, were becoming politically active like never before. They

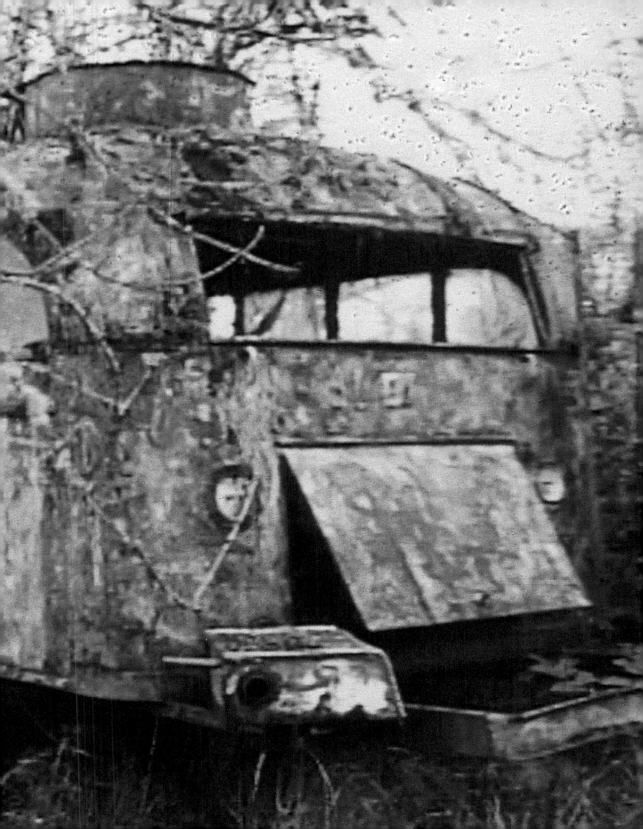

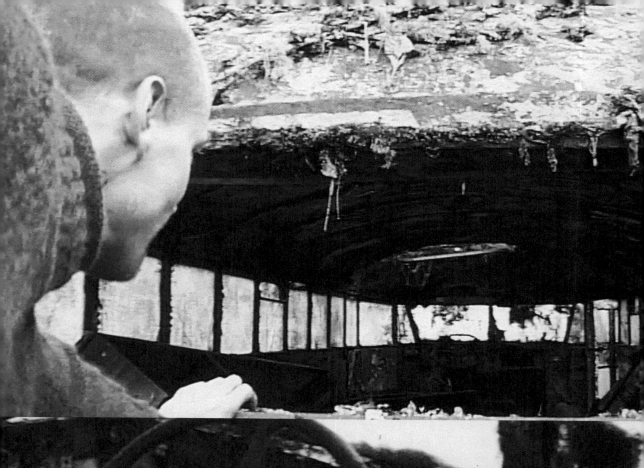

were awake and aware of the problems in society and they weren't afraid to voice themselves.

Thankfully, that's the part of Ken Kesey's legacy that has endured, long after the Merry Pranksters and the pop culture stuff faded away. And we'll never know for sure, but I believe that by helping to shake our society out of a deep sleep, Ken Kesey did succeed, in his own weird way, in stopping the end of the world. For a while anyway.

. . .

The day we met Ken, I remember, we rolled up the long road to his farm just outside of Eugene, Oregon, in the Mothership and found the man himself waiting for us on the porch. I knew from pictures I'd seen of him as a young man that he was a big, strong guy, and he still looked powerful at sixty-seven—like an old prizefighter who had spent a lifetime fighting the good fight. I guess

Ken welcomed each member of our tribe warmly and told us how much he admired and respected what we were trying to do with the SOL Tour. I led him up into the Mothership and took my time showing him around, explaining how all the sustainable systems worked and answering his questions as best I could, just savoring the moment. It was strange at first to be in the presence of someone I'd learned about in high school and college, but Ken was so friendly and interested in our mission that I quickly started to feel like I was with a fellow traveler.

When he finished looking over our mural he motioned with his hand and led us all back into the woods behind the barn. There among the trees, all rusted and almost covered over with vines, sat FURTHER, the Mothership of another generation. Most of the windows were knocked out and the seats had disappeared long ago, but you

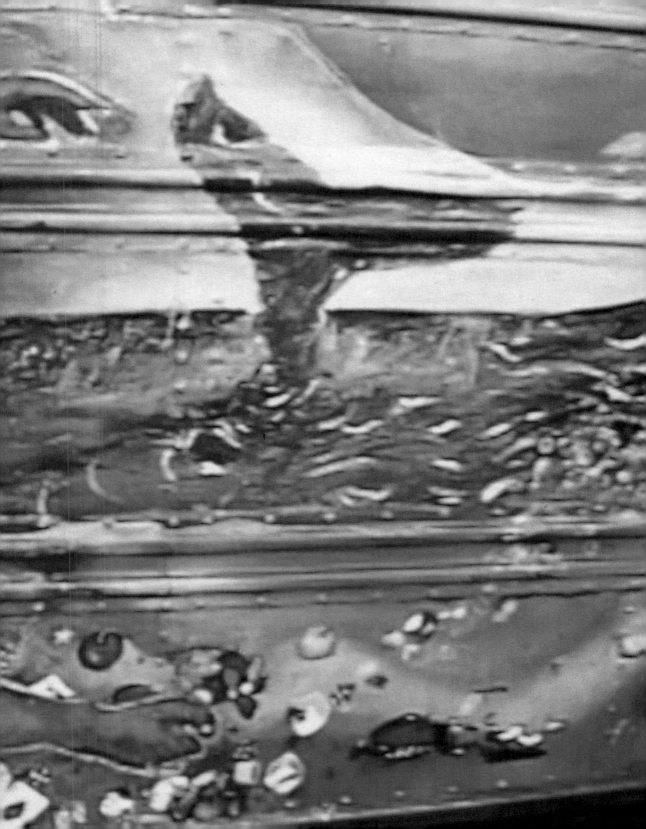

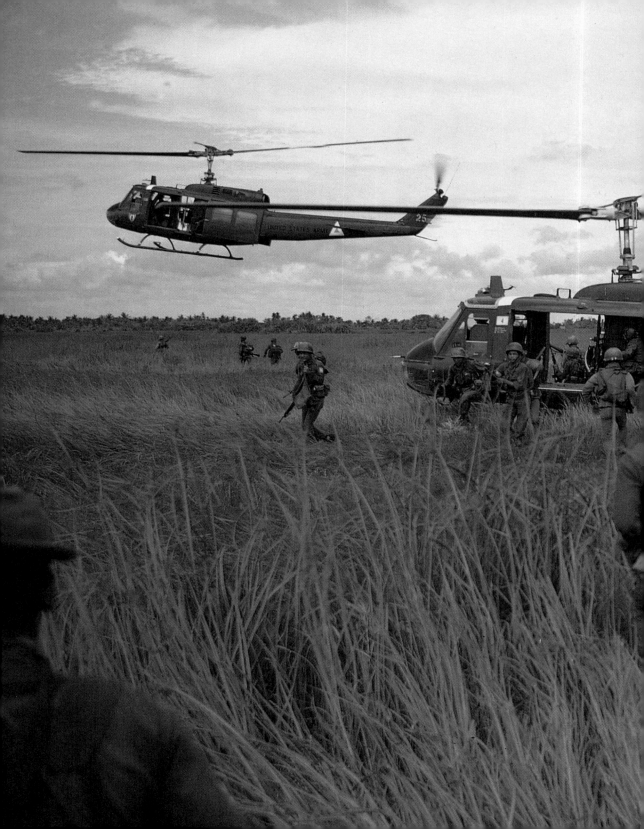

could still see the bright colors of that Day-Glo paintjob lurking under the dirt of years, even decades. Even in that sorry state, that old bus still resonated with history. It was amazing to think that that rusty hulk helped start a movement that marked a generation and changed the world for the better in a lot of ways. You weren't cool in the 60s unless you were "on the bus," and this was the bus everyone was talking about.

We took turns exploring the wreck quietly and respectfully, like you would explore the ruins of a lost civilization. That's exactly how a lot of people look at the 60s today, like some lost relic that has no meaning anymore. But I

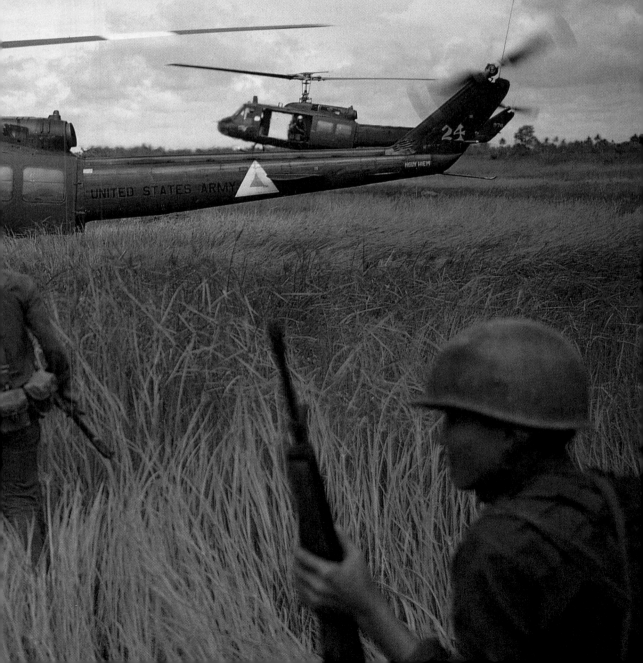

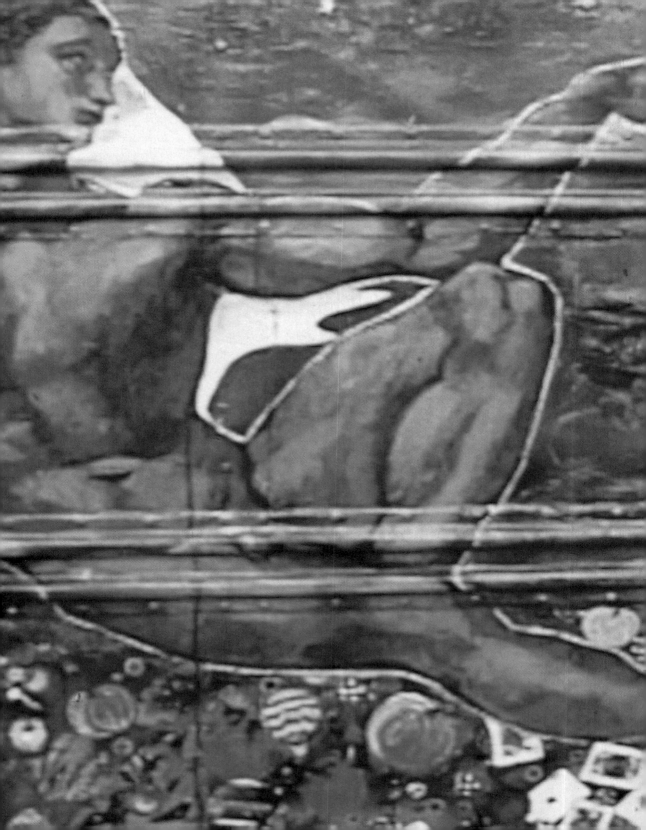

think that couldn't be further from the truth. While it's true that the people who made the 60s such a turning point in history weren't perfect, they still have a lot to be proud of. When it came to things like opposing Vietnam, questioning authority, getting involved politically, and challenging the established norms in society, the hippie generation was right. There's no question about it. And they're still right today.

Unfortunately, in the decades since the 60s, the people who were never "on the bus" have worked very hard to dismiss the idea that anything that came out of that time was ever any good. Mostly it's the people who have a vested interest in society remaining asleep at the wheel—the politicians and the corporations. They point to the world that Ken Kesey feared, the world of the 1950s, as the ideal, when people believed in "family values"—whatever that means—and were fixated on having a house in the suburbs and a nice new car every couple of years. If you're busy keeping up with the Joneses, you stop paying attention to what the people with the power are doing.

In the 60s we were lucky because there were people like Ken who saw the danger and sounded the alarm in any way they could. But we've drifted back off course since then. The question is, who's going to sound the alarm for this generation?

As I picked through the shell of that old bus, the true link between what the Pranksters did almost forty years ago and what we were trying to do on the SOL Tour really hit home for me. The obvious parallel was that we were two groups of true believers traveling around on a bus trying to offer people a living example of other, better, ways to live. But beneath that, there was a more fundamental link, a common goal, and that goal is not necessarily to get people to live like us as much as it is to simply raise their consciousness. The Pranksters used LSD and Day-Glo paint while we used yoga and raw food, but the main idea was the same: there are other ways to live. You should be aware of the alternatives and not be afraid to explore them.

There are still lots of hippies out there, and I know because I met them on the road and saw them at our rallies on the Tour. These weren't hippies in the sense of the Merry Pranksters, with their top hats and painted rocks, but in the sense that they're people who feel they can change the world, and they want to do something about it. Some are old, original hippies who never lost their passion, but most are young and full of the same fire that transformed the FURTHER generation.

When I think about all those eager young faces at our rallies with a sincere desire to walk with a lighter footprint, I realize just how rare an opportunity we had to make a difference. People getting together to talk about changing the world doesn't happen much these days. But if people have the chance to hear about solutions that can improve their life and help the planet, many will embrace them with an incredible energy. It seems to me there are times in history when there's a window of opportunity for society to move in a positive direction. The 60s was obviously one of those times, and a new window is opening now.

I walked away from the old bus with an incredible sense of hope that we could actually make a lasting difference. I had hope because I knew that what we were trying to do was coming from love. It was a love revolution in the 60s and that's what it is now. Why do we want the people we care about to eat right? Because we love them. Why do we want our children to have a clean, healthy world to live in? Because we love them. It's a sweet form of rebellion, and it's effective.

When we left Ken's place, he shook our hands and wished us luck on our journey. He christened us "The Merry Hempsters," and, as he shook my hand, he said that if he were just a few years younger, he'd come along for the ride. I knew he meant it too, but Ken and FURTHER completed their mission long ago; ours was just beginning.

Ken stood and waved as the Mothership moved off down the road, and I looked out the back until we lost sight of him beyond the hills. He died just months later, on November 10, 2001.

• • •

When we began the SOL Tour, we really didn't know what we were getting into. We had some kind of concept that it would be about us going around and talking to people who feel the same way as we do about what needs to happen environmentally, economically, and politically—

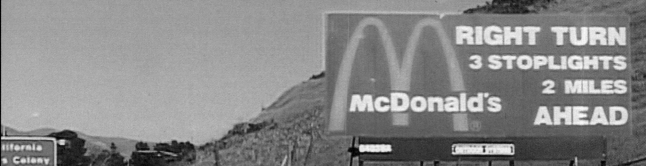

preaching to the choir, really. But as the Tour progressed and we found ourselves speaking to all kinds of individuals, many of whom didn't share our views at all, we realized that we were asking a lot of some people.

It all seemed so simple to us, asking people to evolve and to walk with a lighter footprint on the earth. But then most of the members of our SOL Tour tribe were already there; it was easy for us to talk because we'd already made a transformation in our lives. Then I thought of the people out in the crowd listening to me say, "Personal transformation equals planetary transformation," and thinking to themselves, "I should listen to this guy because he's been in a few movies? How do I know he doesn't drive around Hollywood in an SUV?" It hit me that every time I asked someone else to evolve, my own evolution was equally in question.

The truth is I started out like everybody else, a drug addict. Like every other kid who grew up in America, I started out with the weight-gain drug we call sugar, courtesy of Cap'n Crunch—the ultimate gateway drug if there ever was one. Then they put me on Ritalin because I couldn't sit still in my chair at school. But that's what lots of parents do when they have a kid they can't deal with, right? Don't look for the cause of the behavior, just buy a solution: "Let's give that boy some Ritalin; that'll settle him down."

Before long I was hooked on Coca-Cola, and it felt good. Sugar and caffeine, the corporate speedball. Then I got really hooked on that totally fucked-up drug called McDonald's. By the time I was in my twenties I was a complete mess, hooked on the best government-approved corporate drugs money could buy. Looking back on that time in my life now, I can say with confidence that the corporate drugs are a lot more destructive than some of the illegal ones they spend billions of our tax dollars trying to fight.

I was a corporate drug junkie but I don't feel any shame in that because for most of my life I didn't have anyone to show me a better way. Besides, the corporate drugs felt good, and everybody does them; that's why they're so hard to kick. I didn't realize at the time, though, that you can never get enough of the corporate drugs. They're designed to work like that: the more you have, the more you want.

So while I had my sugar and my caffeine and my saturated fat to meet my internal needs, I had the pursuit of the American Dream to meet all my external needs. I admit it: I always wanted to be rich and famous. Who doesn't? And when I achieved that goal I made the most of it, living out all the fantasies and indulging in all the excesses. But after a while I started to notice that the pursuit of things left me feeling the same as the corporate drugs: empty.

One of the perks of being in movies is that you get to meet a lot of famous people. I've met a lot of people with immense success and lots of money and fame, and I found that few, if any, are very happy. They're unhappy because they're looking for external things to fill them up, and it doesn't work. I know that was true of me. In fact, it's often the most successful people who feel the emptiest, like political leaders and the heads of all these

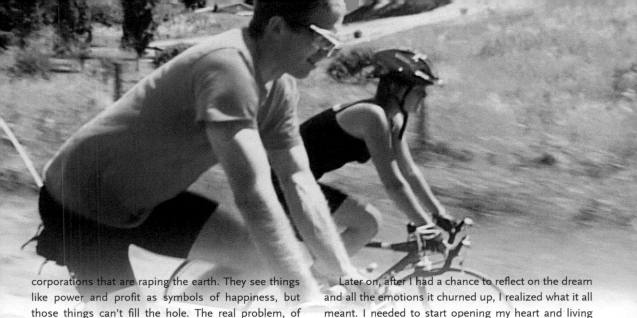

corporations that are raping the earth. They see things like power and profit as symbols of happiness, but those things can't fill the hole. The real problem, of course, is that they don't have any love in their heart.

That's really when the transformation started for me—when I finally figured out that it isn't about money or fame or stuff; it's about love. And really, what needs to happen in the world more than anything is an evolution of the heart, and that evolution has to start within each individual.

I'll be the first to admit that for a long time my heart was closed off to the world. I worked hard to put up emotional moats and fences and barbwire to keep people at a distance. I used to say I did it to keep myself from getting hurt, but now I know that I really did it so I could ignore all the negative shit about myself that i didn't want to look at—like how my diet was killing me and my greed was killing me and how I was sleepwalking through my life. I just didn't want to look—really look—inside myself and demand some change.

They say addicts usually don't commit to making positive changes in their life until they hit rock bottom. Well, rock bottom came for me one night in the form of a horrible dream. I dreamed that a very close friend of mine was killed, and I spent the rest of the dream trying to avenge his death. The dream went on all night, and even when I tried to wake up from it I couldn't. It was a terrible night, and it left me feeling physically drained and shaken up emotionally. The next day I got up and called my friend right away to make sure he was OK and to let him know how much I cared about him.

Later on, after I had a chance to reflect on the dream and all the emotions it churned up, I realized what it all meant. I needed to start opening my heart and living with love, or I would never be happy. That evolution starts with loving yourself, by taking care of your body by eating right and exercising, then extends out to touch your family and friends. It can't stop there though; if you want to really transform your life you have to make an effort to love your fellow humans and love the planet. You do that by taking responsibility for the choices you make as a consumer and as a citizen of the world.

Once I understood that, and I mean really got it, that's when things started to change for the better in my life where it really matters—physically and emotionally. My heart was completely open for the first time, and I started to live with real love, for myself, my family and friends, but also for people in general and the earth as well.

Once I was committed to my personal evolution, I simply would not allow my heart to be closed off anymore. It couldn't be, not if I wanted to be a part of the big evolution, or revolution, that I believe needs to happen for the planet to survive. Because when we allow ourselves to get stuck in patterns that aren't any good for us and aren't any good for anybody else either, what's really happening is that we are closing off our heart. But I believe the natural state of a human being is to be loving, and nurturing, and considerate. Unfortunately, we spend a lot of time trying to force ourselves into an unnatural state, whether it's with bad food or corporate drugs or greed. Evolving personally is about letting go of all the

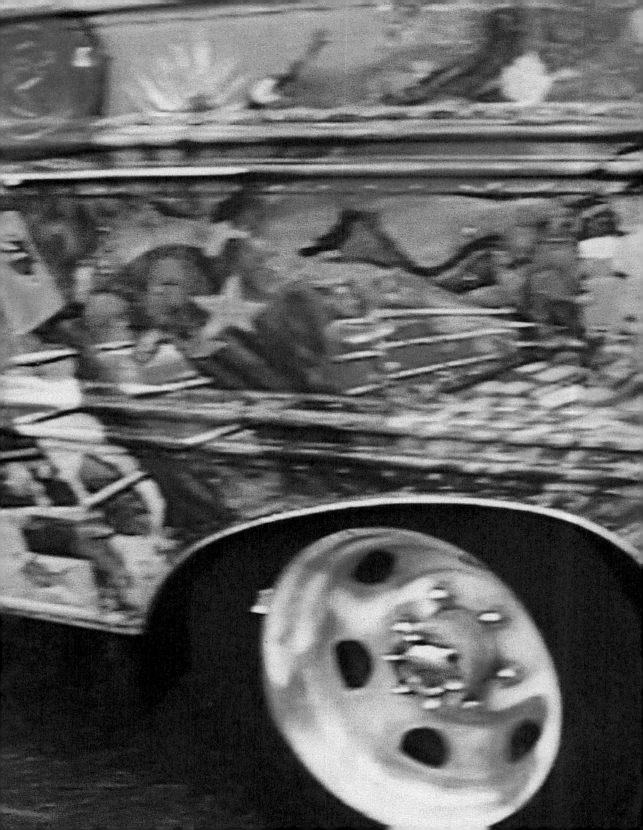

unnatural crap in your life and getting back to that natural, healthy, loving state.

It's taken me a while, but that's where I believe I am at right now. My heart is wide open, and I try every day to do all I can to love myself the way I should and to treat the people around me and the earth with love, as well. But it's also a commitment I have to make every day. That's the frame of mind I brought to the SOL Tour, but I had to be clear on that before I could feel comfortable asking other people to evolve.

Almost every day on the SOL Tour, I would find myself in front of a group of people saying, "Please feel enough for yourself and for the earth to think about the consequences of your personal actions and maybe just try to shift a little in the right direction each day." After I said that, in my head I would always ask myself, "But am I shifting?" And every day, I'm happy to say, the answer was "yes." The answer is still "yes."

• • •

The hardest part of any journey is just getting started, and the journey of personal evolution is no different. When I was out on the road asking people to evolve, I noticed that just the thought of making a change in their lives was enough to make some of them pull back. I could almost see them locking their heart up in their personal safe deposit box for protection.

The funny thing is, I also found that most people out there already have some sense that the world is dealing with some major issues, and many of them already know that they need to make changes in their diet to become healthier. It's like the seeds for all of the ideas we were talking about on the SOL Tour— eating organic, doing yoga, living sustainably, consumer responsibility—had already been planted. Those seeds just needed a bit of watering and attention to start growing. So our challenge was not so much introducing people to these ideas as it was inspiring them to act on stuff they'd already been thinking about.

So many people are so stuck in their negative patterns, the only way for them to start a personal transformation is to try to step outside themselves and look at their life from a distance. When I spoke at rallies on the SOL Tour, I often asked the people who came to think about themselves and analyze every aspect of their lives—the food they eat, the clothes they wear, the power they consume, the products they buy, the politicians they support. Essentially, everyone's life breaks down into a series of choices, and it's possible for people to look at the choices they make and determine the kind of impact each choice has on themselves personally, on society and on the environment.

Once you go through that exercise of pulling back from your life and really looking at the impact of the choices you make, an amazing thing happens: You start to see yourself as a part of the environment, because you know you have the power to harm it. Instead of closing yourself off in your own little world, you start to think about your place in the whole world, and that changes you. Soon, the layers of crap you don't need start to dissolve as you begin to question each choice you make. And when that happens, you're on your way to personal transformation.

It is important to remember, though, that evolving is never easy. In fact, it's very difficult, and it gets much more difficult before it gets any easier. It can be emotional, and it takes a lot of energy to stay committed to change. Basically, you have to assess the values you've been living with and decide which ones to throw out and which ones to keep, and that's never easy, especially if you've been living for years with the same self-destructive values. We were asking people to move from one complete state of mind to another, but we never said the whole journey was going to be smooth and enjoyable.

A lot of people just can't do it, because it's so much easier to stay where they're comfortable, even if it's killing them and making things worse for everyone else. But that's the trade-off: there's a price to pay for anything good in life, and in order to feel better about yourself and how you're living, you often have to endure some kind of pain. In fact, just to be open to change is hard, because any time you open yourself up you feel vulnerable. But vulnerability is essential if you want to evolve; it's that vulnerability that opens you up to learning about the alternatives.

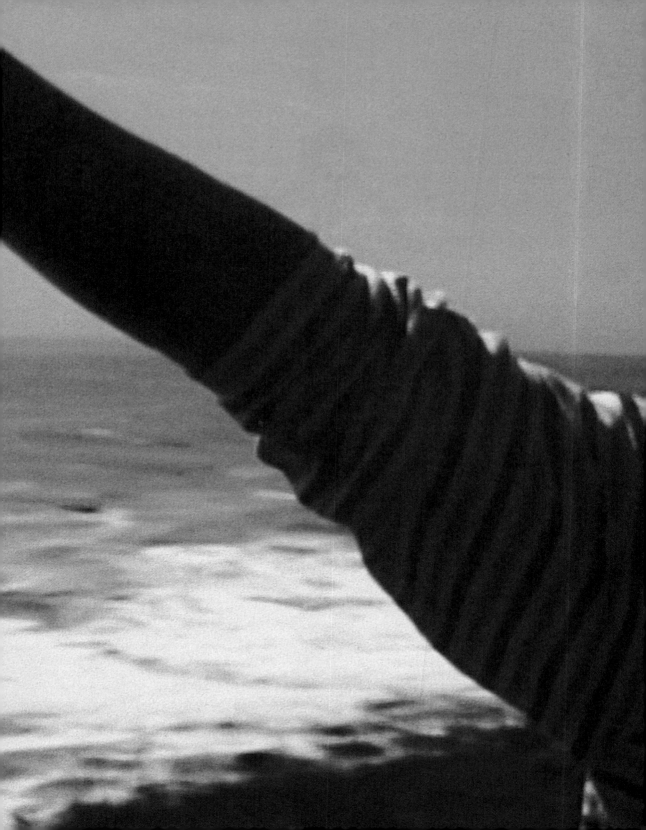

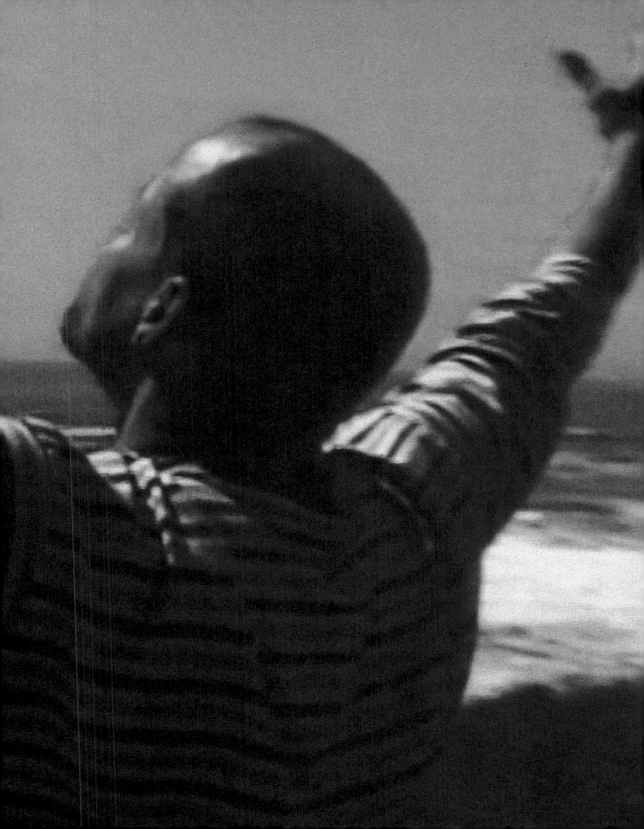

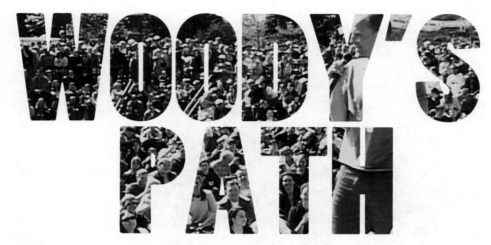

WOODY'S PATH

When I spoke to groups during the SOL Tour, I would tell little stories about my personal evolution that sort of illustrated my key points. One story I liked to tell in particular was about a funny little incident that helped me to really understand the current situation we find ourselves in on this planet.

A few years back, I was in Hawaii visiting with friends and we decided to take a walk down to this beautiful rainwater pool nearby and have a swim. The spot— Emerald Pool I think it's called—is like a hidden tropical paradise in the middle of a palm forest. It's fed by a stream of water running down from the hillside and over a volcanic rock waterfall. We spent a wonderful afternoon there, just diving into the crystal-clear rainwater and drying off in the bright Hawaiian sun. A perfect day, except for one little incident.

At one end of the pool there was a rock, perfectly flat and just right for one person to stretch out on and soak up the sun. As soon as I spotted it, naturally, I swam right over and made myself comfortable. With the sun beating down, I had just settled into a nice euphoric state when I felt something big and wet and hairy scramble up beside me. It was my friend's dog, Wookie. Apparently Wookie had been swimming at Emerald Pool before and she had had her eye on that nice flat rock as well.

The feel of Wookie's wet dog butt on my leg was definitely taking away from the whole experience, but I

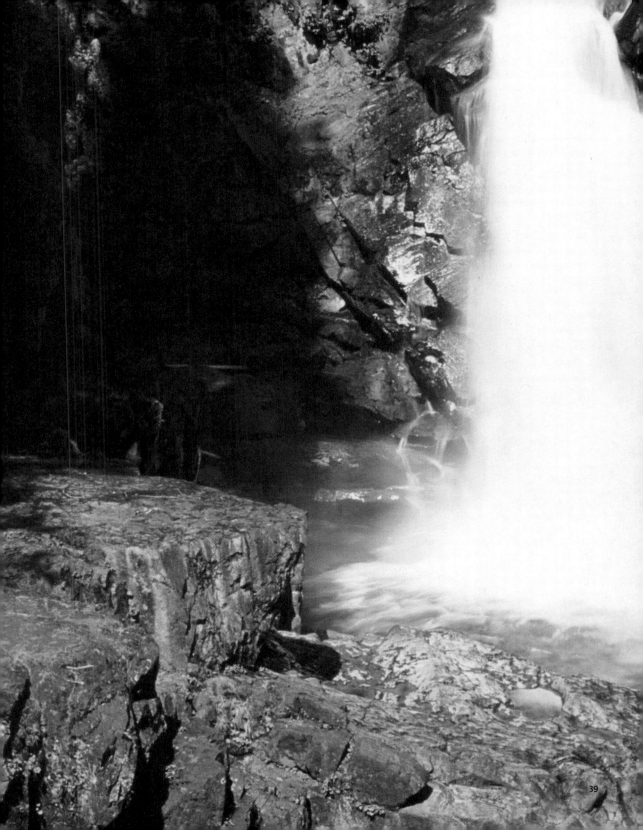

figured, "OK Wookie, I can share." I scooted over a few inches to give her some room to sit down, but sitting was not what Wookie had in mind. As dogs are wont to do when they come out of the water, Wookie put her head down and shook as hard as she possibly could, transferring just about every drop of water on her fur to my body. I leaned away to try to protect myself and in the process I gave up another few inches of rock to Wookie. She immediately saw her opportunity and laid down right across the rock, pushing her butt back up against my back. I tried to scoot over again, but I ran out of room and slipped right back into the water.

My buddy looked over and started laughing at me: "Woody, what happened to your rock?"

"I guess it's Wookie's rock now," I said, shaking my head. That pretty girl just closed her eyes and settled in for some serious sunbathing; she sure as hell wasn't going anywhere.

That experience with Wookie the dog was just a funny little experience, but I thought about it later on and it occurred to me that the same thing is happening every day all over the world on a much larger, and much more sinister, scale. I made room for Wookie because I didn't realize she wanted the whole rock, and she was just doing what came naturally. But when you think about it, that's kind of the same way the large corporations get control of things; we let them have their way in exchange for creating jobs and obeying the law and paying taxes, then once we become dependent on them, they stop doing those things. The scary thing is, our perfect rock is the earth, and I believe we the people are being "Wookied" off that rock.

There's no doubt in my mind that there are forces working hard to take our planet away inch by inch, because I've seen the evidence. As we cycled down through the Northwest, we passed acres and acres of clear-cut where, since the dawn of time, lush forests had once stood and nurtured hundreds of species of wildlife. I wondered how many of those trees were destroyed to make paper so the brokers on Wall Street could keep track of their stocks. Half the trees cut down in the U.S. every year are used to make paper, even

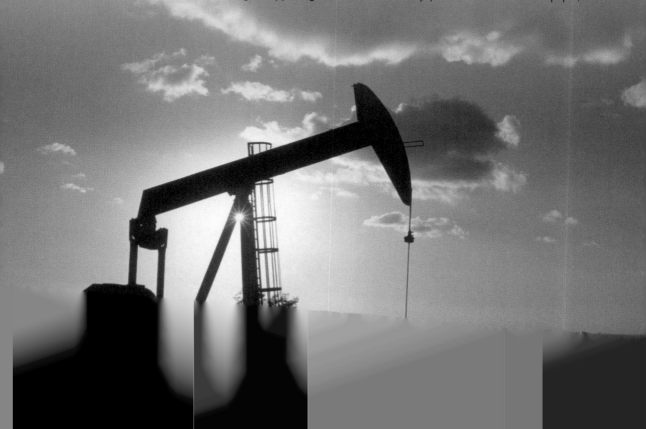

though we know we don't need to make paper from trees. That's a couple of inches off the rock right there.

Then you look at where most of our energy comes from: non-sustainable fossil fuels that create choking smog and pollute the landscape. Cotton for clothing is grown with the help of millions of gallons of deadly pesticides. What used to be just vegetables on our dinner plate are now genetically modified, copyrighted products grown by a chemical company. And the government? Well, the politicians who are supposed to protect us from getting Wookied off our rock can't even begin to get elected without the backing of big business, so don't look to them for help. It doesn't have to be this way, of course; the alternatives are right in front of us. But still we continue to buy whatever the corporations throw at us and go on giving up more and more space on our rock in the process.

We can't blame it all on corporate greed though; to a large extent, we've allowed this to happen. By its very design, our consumer-driven society forces us into separate groups based on our ability to buy. Ads on TV and in magazines tell us that if we consume more—have a bigger house, drive a bigger SUV, eat a bigger steak—we'll stand out from our neighbors, as if being better customers somehow makes us better people. Of course, that's only a myth perpetrated by the forces trying to Wookie us off our rock. It creates people who are separate from each other and separate from the natural world. And if you're separate, you're a hell of a lot easier to deal with. "That's right," they say, "just keep wearing that suit and punching that clock, making somebody else's dreams come true." See, if you're just a cog in the machine, you're much more likely to approve when the machine does something destructive.

But why do we do it? Why do we let those forces take another inch of our rock when we have the power to stop them? I'm sorry to say that a lot of it has to do with our own greed. Many people in the world today have bought into the advertisers' notion that more is always better, to the point where even the people who already have too much want even more. The concept of wealth has been twisted to refer only to consumer wealth, as if

Genetic Modification

Genetically Modified Organisms, or GMOs, are created by moving genes from species to species. GMOs are created in the laboratory by taking bacterial enzymes from one organism, cutting out specific genetic markers, and splicing their DNA into a second organism. During this process, the genes are duplicated many times and are turned into small copies of themselves. Rings in the DNA, called plasmids, move the DNA from one species to the other. Creating GMOs is not an easy task, and currently only small amounts of an organism's cells can be successfully altered.

Until midway through the 1990s, consumers were unable to tell whether or not they were buying genetically modified food because scientists were unable to tell with accuracy whether or not a given organism had been genetically modified. Since then, new methods have been developed to help scientists determine whether or not food is genetically modified. However, few jurisdictions in North America require that these foods be labeled as GMOs.

Research has indicated that genetically engineered plants are twenty times more likely to interbreed with non-genetically engineered plants. And crops that are modified to produce pharmaceuticals cross-breeding with non-genetically engineered plants could contaminate the ecosystem and expose animals to drugs that could kill them. —KH.

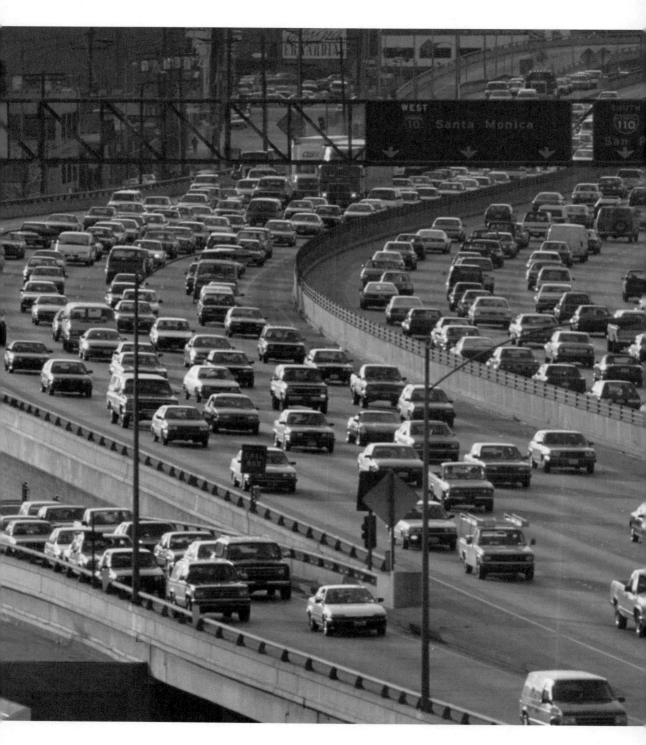

things like wealth of experience and wealth of love and wealth of good health had no value at all. A lot of people are on autopilot these days, consuming without knowing why, never asking themselves the good questions like, "Why am I ordering a double burger and Biggie fries at the drive-thru at 11:00 at night?"

The good news is, we can still stop ourselves from being Wookied off our rock, and the solution is simple. I'm not talking about violent protest or a march on the capital or anything drastic like that, although I do believe those things have their time and place. But if there's one word that scares the forces trying to take control of this planet more than any other, it's *sustainability*. Sustainability is a dangerous concept because when consumers focus on sustainability—meaning they actually stop and think about every dollar they spend—the spell is broken and they get a chance to clear their heads. And it's when people start to see the world with clear eyes that they begin to see alternatives. It won't take much to stop the slide either; if we all scale back on our wants just a little bit, I bet that'd do it. Then from moderation we can begin the shift to sustainability. That's when we start pushing in the opposite direction, and begin to take our rock back.

So what exactly are these forces slowly taking over the planet, tree by tree, farm by farm, and wildlife preserve by wildlife preserve? We all know the names—the Nikes, the Monsantos, the Weyerhaeusers, the Halliburtons—they permeate every aspect of our lives. Mining, petroleum, timber, nuclear, pharmaceuticals, and agribusiness industries feast on billions of dollars in subsidies from the government. It's a long list for sure, but for the sake of clarity, I just refer to the whole bunch of them as "the Beast." These are the corporations that, with the help of organizations like the World

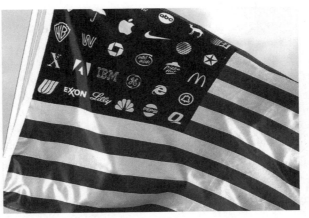

Trade Organization (WTO) and the World Bank, control the economy of the entire world and are threatening to Wookie us right off our rock. I know it's easy to feel powerless in the face of such a massive force, but we can take it down if we all do what we can in unified fashion. We won't kill this beast with one blow; it's too big and strong. But we just might get it with the death by a thousand cuts.

The first thing you need to understand is that the Beast is everywhere, and it has an enormous appetite that is never satisfied. So the first step in walking with a lighter footprint on the earth is making the connection between what you consume and how the Beast gets fed, because the Beast only bothers with people who are willing to sustain it. Do you drive a big SUV to work when you could use public transit? Mark of the Beast. Do you use a couple of paper towels instead of a cloth to wipe some water off the coffee table? Mark of the Beast. Do you put one wet item in the dryer for fifteen minutes instead of hanging it on the clothesline? Beast again. Do you clean with products like Windex, Palmolive, Tide? Most commercial cleansers and detergents are a thousand times more toxic than anything not "clean."

It really is amazing where you find the mark of the Beast when you start to think about the way you live your life. Things you use every day and don't even think about, like shampoo and conditioner, often have petroleum byproducts in them. Organic shampoos wash your hair just as well without the crude, and they don't feed the Beast. Think of the journey that paper cup from the water cooler had to make to get from the forest to your hand just to have you take one drink out of it and throw it in the garbage can. Is rinsing a glass out

The World Bank and the World Trade Organization

• Under the leadership of the U.S. and British governments, the International Bank for Reconstruction and Development was set up after World War II to provide loans for post-war reconstruction in Europe. Later known as the World Bank, its purpose shifted in the 1950s to funding industrial projects in developing countries. In the decades since, many of these countries have incurred huge debts. The World Bank and the International Monetary Fund (IMF) have used this debt-load as leverage to demand certain economic adjustments, such as deregulation, privatization of publicly owned enterprises, and curbs on budget deficits in these countries. These measures have often led to fewer social and educational programs, greater pollution, and higher poverty levels in the affected countries.

• The General Agreement on Tariffs and Trade (GATT) was established in 1947 to create and enforce multilateral trade agreements. In 1995, the World Trade Organization (WTO) was founded as the successor to the GATT. In the 1990s, the WTO became the focal point for public debate over the effects of economic globalization: many fear that in the globalization process the interests of transnational corporations are being permitted to override the interests of local populations, particularly in the areas of human rights, labor laws, and pollution regulations.

Sources: Manfred B. Steger, Globalization; David Ransom, The No-Nonsense Guide to Fair Trade.

once a day really such a chore? Mark of the Beast.

That's how it started for me. When I decided I wanted to walk with a lighter footprint, I started to look at how I was living and I made a conscious effort to make changes: turning off lights during the day, looking for ways to use less paper and plastic. As I got more and more into the process, I actually started to get a kick out of pushing back against the Beast. I remember being in a grocery store one time and the cashier asked me, "Paper or plastic?"

With a big grin I held up my hemp grocery bag and said, "Neither, thanks."

Of course, you can't evolve if you don't make a commitment to be completely honest with yourself. You know as an individual how heavy your footprint is on the earth. You know as an individual how much you do to feed the Beast. I know, I've been there: speeding down the road in my convertible Corvette, drinking Coca-Cola from a Styrofoam cup, air-conditioner blasting. It's times like that when you have to be honest and ask yourself, "Am I doing all I can?" Because if you can't address what's going on with you, you can't begin to address what's going on in the world.

But that's not to say that there's only one right way to evolve. I'm not presenting the concept of walking with a lighter footprint as a black or white, right or wrong proposition. The SOL Tour was about a bunch of people trying to lead their lives in a way that they believe is a better, safer, cleaner, kinder way to exist. But we never tried to present ourselves as a perfect model for everyone else to emulate. I believe that the way I choose to live my life now is more considerate,

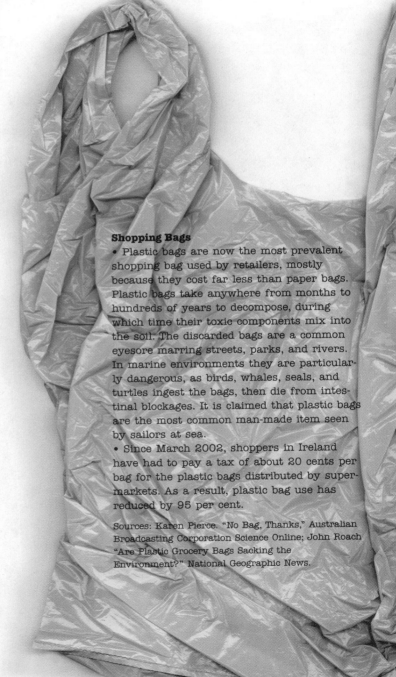

Shopping Bags

• Plastic bags are now the most prevalent shopping bag used by retailers, mostly because they cost far less than paper bags. Plastic bags take anywhere from months to hundreds of years to decompose, during which time their toxic components mix into the soil. The discarded bags are a common eyesore marring streets, parks, and rivers. In marine environments they are particularly dangerous, as birds, whales, seals, and turtles ingest the bags, then die from intestinal blockages. It is claimed that plastic bags are the most common man-made item seen by sailors at sea.

• Since March 2002, shoppers in Ireland have had to pay a tax of about 20 cents per bag for the plastic bags distributed by supermarkets. As a result, plastic bag use has reduced by 95 per cent.

Sources: Karen Pierce. "No Bag, Thanks," Australian Broadcasting Corporation Science Online; John Roach "Are Plastic Grocery Bags Sacking the Environment?" National Geographic News.

TV

Number of leisure hours the average
American has per week: 35

Number of hours the average
American spends watching TV per
week: 28

Source: Steger, <u>Globalization,</u> p.72

kind, and ultimately fulfilling than the way I lived in the past. But no, it's not perfect. When I started my transformation, I don't think I believed I could incorporate some of the changes I've made into my life. But I was open to the ideas and made the changes I could, in my own way and at my own pace. That's all we ever asked anyone to do: be open, be curious, be inquisitive, ask questions. If you look, you can find other ways to do things.

Ultimately, it's up to each individual to decide how far he or she is going to shift, but every little bit helps. I think the most important thing is just to have an open mind when it comes to looking at the alternatives. Think about them for even just ten seconds longer than you would do naturally. Then, after you've taken the time to explore the different ways you can live a more sustainable lifestyle, determine which ones you can apply to your daily life and which ones don't work for you. I don't believe there is anyone out there, certainly not in the developed world, who can't find any possible way to walk with a lighter footprint. If there is, I'd love to meet them, because I could definitely learn a lot. Even actor Ed Begley, Jr., an environmentalist I greatly admire and who truly walks his talk, could probably make *some* changes.

But probably the greatest thing about opening your mind up to new ideas about how to live a simpler, healthier lifestyle is that it's so empowering. We've been socialized to think that our choices are always limited to what the Beast provides: Nike or Adidas, Shell or Exxon, McDonald's or Burger King, Democrat or Republican. But when you get active and involved in changing your life and actually go out and investigate the alternatives, you will find that there is, in fact, a column C, and that's where most of the good stuff is. Once you know that, you don't have to accept the reality they hand you on TV or in the magazine ads anymore. Once you know there's another way, you can think for yourself and follow your own path. Guess what? You really don't have to keep giving money to the Beast so he can hold your mother hostage. How cool is that?

I really do believe that the time has come to shake the Etch-a-Sketch, and my experiences on the SOL Tour tell me that a lot of other people feel the same way. If we can just get all those people working on their own individual evolution, I know we can achieve a huge collective change for the good. And I truly believe that moving toward sustainability is the way to go.

Much of the time, the activism you see is really reactivism, where we see something wrong and we say, "Hey, this has got to stop," then we react: we hold protests or sit-ins, we shut down an intersection, we shut down a city. Shit, in Seattle we managed to shut

Globalization: social processes of intensifying global interdependence. **Globalism:** an ideology that associates the concept of globalization with neoliberal values such as free trade, privatization, deregulation, tax cuts, and controls on organized labor.

Source: Steger, Globalization.

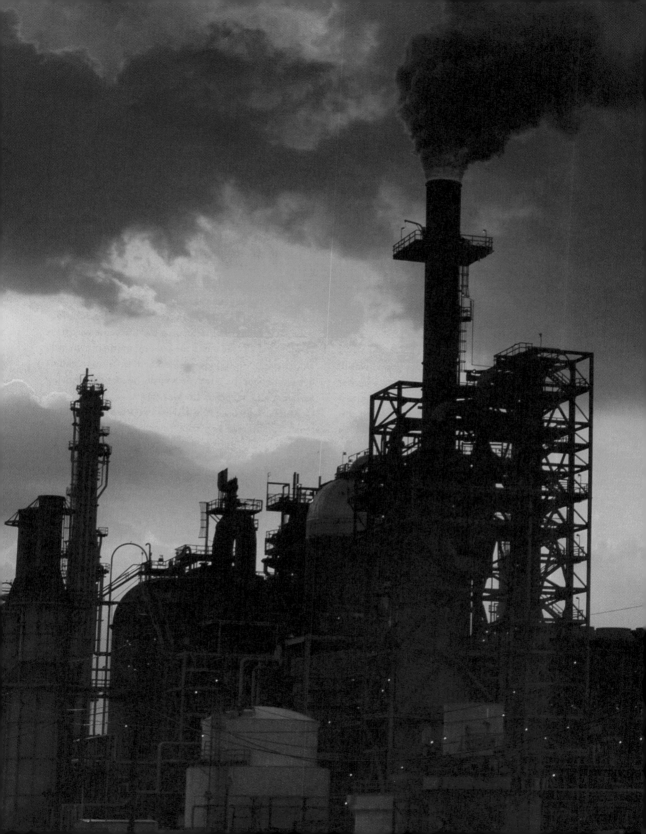

down the WTO. But I see that kind of activism as only a fifty per cent solution, because you're constantly on the defensive, just trying to plug holes in the dike. Moving toward sustainability, on the other hand, is proactive, because this way you're saying, "Here's something right; this is the way to go." You force the Beast to react to you, and that's a one hundred per cent solution.

You could call Simple Organic Living a new social

from time to time, split up into many smaller streams. But any time there's a crisis, our various streams always seem to find a way to come together to form a river. And I think we're at a time now when there's a great confluence happening, where environmentalists, social justice activists, civil rights activists, Fair Trade activists, and the labor movement are coming together and trying to build understanding and unity. And we need it, there's no

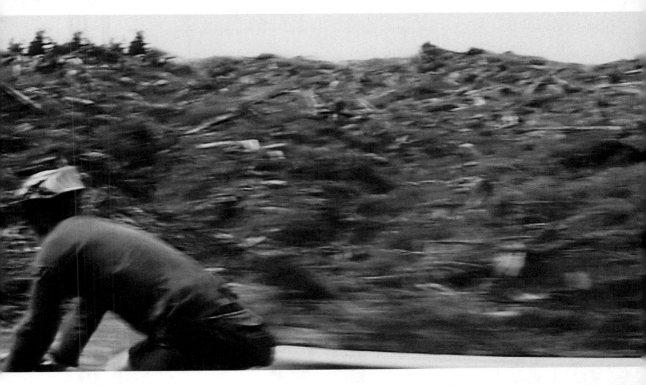

movement, but are any of them new? Down through the centuries, motivated individuals have had to come together at various times to fight for positive change. The enemy always had a different name but its goal was always the same: world domination. We've already seen the evils of imperialism, colonialism, fascism, capitalism; now we're struggling with globalism.

So did the "movement" ever go away, or at least the natural desire of decent people to resist the forces of domination? I don't think so. I think we've been fractured

doubt—because it's going to take a lot of creative thought and effective action to get this Beast off our rock.

For the most part, the people I encountered on the SOL Tour were open to the idea of walking with a lighter footprint. But, at the same time, I also encountered a lot of people who would listen to our message of sustainability, then look me straight in the eye and say, "Hey, I'm comfortable. I obey the law and pay my taxes. Why should I bother?" That attitude always left me at a loss for words; I mean how do you reach out to those who feel so disconnected from their fellow humans and from nature that they believe their personal actions have no effect on anyone but themselves? And how do you convince them to walk with a lighter footprint on the earth when they won't even admit the earth has a problem? The scientific community has been telling us for years about the dangers of pollution, pesticides, toxic waste, global warming, and the abuse of our natural resources, yet there are still people out there who simply choose to ignore it.

Personally, I don't know how those people do it. I don't know how someone can look at a clear-cut forest and not admit that the environment is deteriorating rapidly under the impact of human activity. I don't know how someone can see a family member suffering from heart disease or cancer and not admit that negative lifestyle choices have an impact on your health. And I don't know how anyone could believe that we *Homo sapiens* were designed by nature to eat food created in a laboratory. For me, all of these issues are linked; there's an undeniable connection between what we eat and the way we consume and the well-being of both ourselves and the environment.

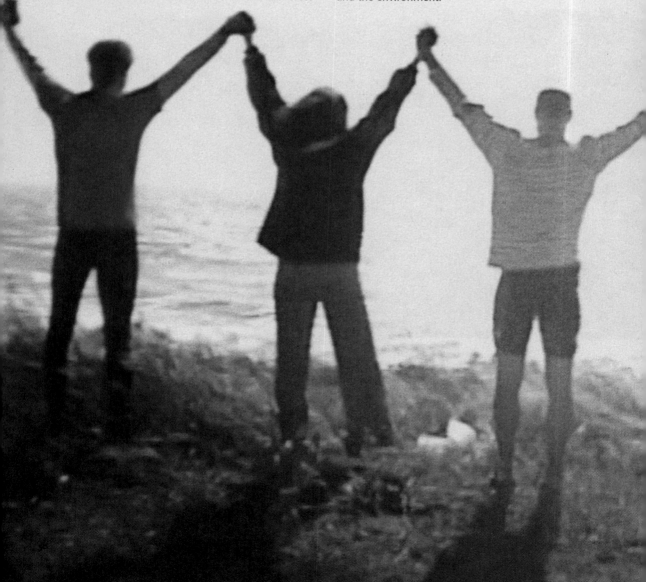

Still, I can't let people who don't want to change stop my evolution; I've got too much at stake. Just like everybody else, I've only got so much time to make a statement with my life, and the question is, is that statement going to be the one I want to make? Is it going to be a statement that is in alignment with what I believe inside? I want to know when I'm done that I stood for something, and that it was something that was right for me and right for the world. And if I ever lose sight of that, all I have to do is look into my kids' eyes and I'll get all the inspiration I need to keep going.

I often ended my little talks on the Tour by asking the people in the crowd to answer two questions. First, do you think the world needs changing? And, assuming you do think the world needs changing, how would you go about changing it? The thing is, it might seem like there are lots of different answers to the second question, but the fact is there really is only one right answer: change yourself first. That's it. Become your own ideal, the ideal that you want to see in the world around you. Then other people will see you evolving and want to know what you're doing—that's how you change the world.

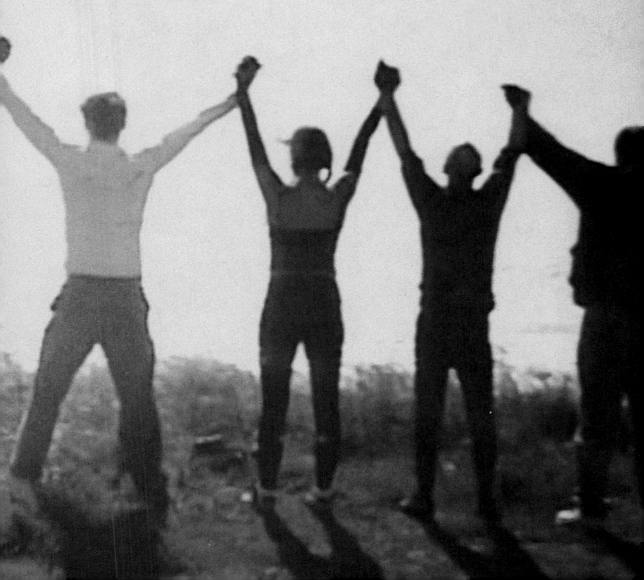

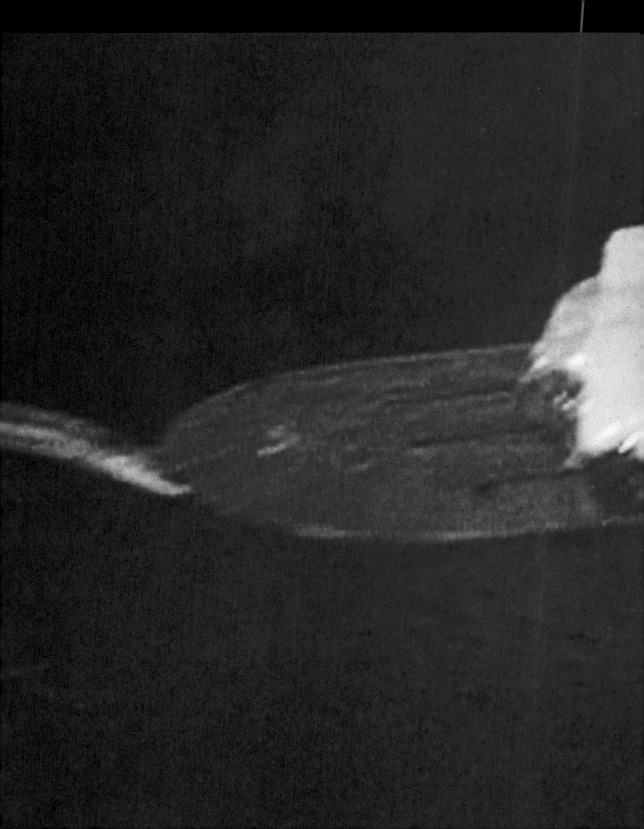

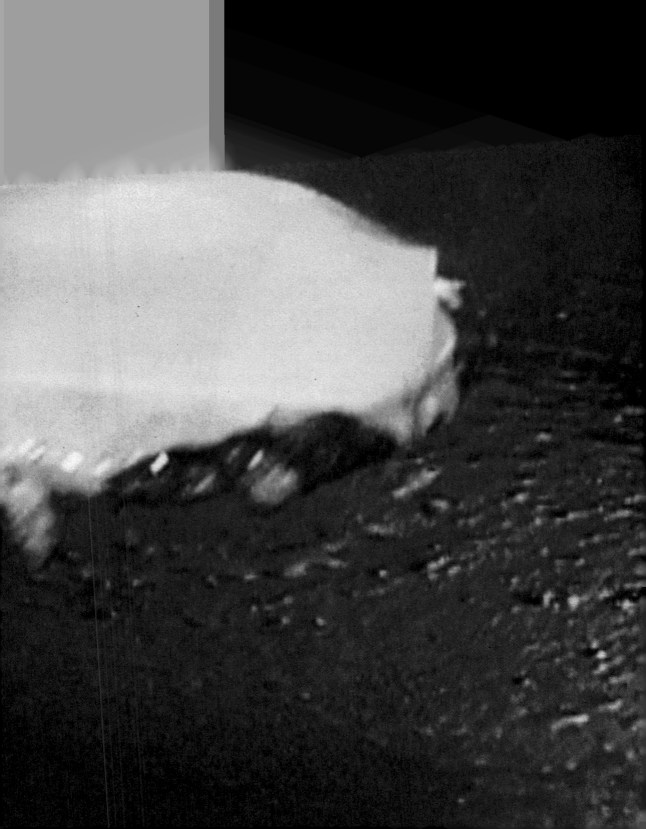

DIET

One of the most important lessons that I've learned in my life—one that took me a long time to learn—is that personal transformation equals planetary transformation.

Lots of people talk about wanting to change the planet, and many even make an honest effort to do it, either by working to change their government, save the environment, eliminate poverty, or maybe protest globalization. While I agree that we really do need to do those kinds of things, I've come to believe that the easiest way to change the planet, in ways that you can measure today, is to take a good hard look at your own life and figure out what positive changes you can make there, starting with what you eat.

Becoming a vegan was probably the biggest change I ever made in my life, and one of my greatest accomplishments as well. It was a real struggle in the beginning, but now I'm proud to say that I eat a totally plant-based diet—no meat, no dairy, one hundred per cent organic (that's a top priority), and the fresher the food, the better. I wish I could say I ate an "all raw food" diet, but I don't. I probably eat about ninety per cent raw, but I still let a little dead food slip in there now and again. At least I'm moving in the right direction.

For me, changing my diet was a personal transformation that has touched every aspect of my life, and I'm reaping the benefits today in terms of my health, my personal relationships, and my relationship with the planet. But that transformation didn't happen overnight—far from it. I had to struggle with junk food withdrawal and re-learn everything I thought I knew about food and nutrition before I managed to get myself on the right path. Weaning yourself off

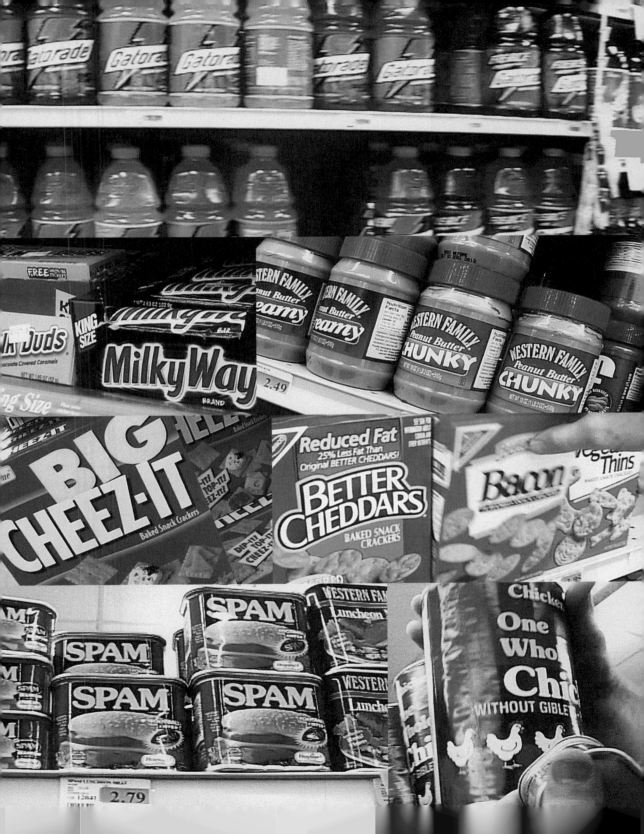

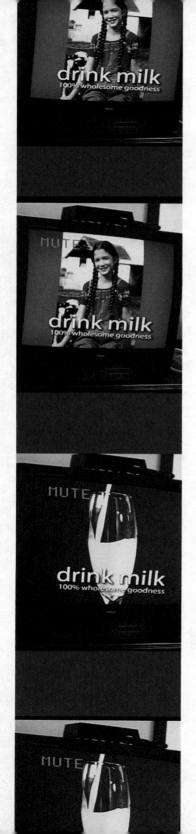

the sugar and fat teat is hard, I know, especially when you're young and you still think your body is invincible. But it's never too early, or too late, to learn the most important diet lesson of them all: the road to an early grave runs right through your mouth.

When I started on the road to my personal transformation, I was living a life that most people would find pretty familiar, except that I was probably a little more excessive than most about my bad habits. I was about twenty-three years old—I liked my Coke, and my Twinkies and my glazed donuts, and they knew me by name down at the McDonald's drive-thru. I actually thought I was doing myself a favor by drinking milk, because the commercials on TV were telling me, "Milk does a body good," and I bought it, just like everybody else. Of course, I didn't waste any time at all back then thinking about how my choices might affect other people or the environment; I was just a young, self-centered guy thinking about my career and being successful and having fun—and I did have a lot of that.

Health-wise, your body can put up with a lot of bullshit when you're a kid and a young adult, especially if you're as active as I was, playing basketball and working out. It's like you can eat all kinds of crap but you don't seem to gain weight and your energy level is always high. Sooner or later though, all that fat and refined sugar catches up with you, no matter how much time you spend in the gym.

I guess I was a pretty healthy-looking specimen when I was in my early twenties, from the outside at least. I had a fairly athletic physique and a nice tan from the California sun. Hell, I still had most of my hair. When I look back on it now though, there were signs there that my body was trying to tell me something.

First of all, the whole time I was growing up I had what you might call a chronic runny nose. It didn't matter whether I had a cold or not, my head was always full of mucus and I was always blowing my nose and trying to clear my head so I could breathe properly. On top of the snot, I also fought an ongoing battle with acne and blotches of red discoloration on my skin. Some times were worse than others, but the symptoms would always come back no matter what I did. I went to doctors and specialists to try and figure out what the problem was and they gave me pills to clear my sinuses and creams for my skin, but all their fixes were only ever temporary. In the end, it was a complete stranger who gave me the answer to my problem, and ended up changing the course of my life at the same time.

One day, I got on the bus to go somewhere and I sat down beside a girl about my age who had her nose buried in a book. It wasn't long before the mucus started to build up, and pretty soon I was snorting and coughing and blowing my nose, making all kinds of nasty noises. She was pretty good about it for about ten minutes; she just kept on reading her book and pretending she couldn't hear me. Eventually, though, I guess she couldn't take it anymore and looked up at me.

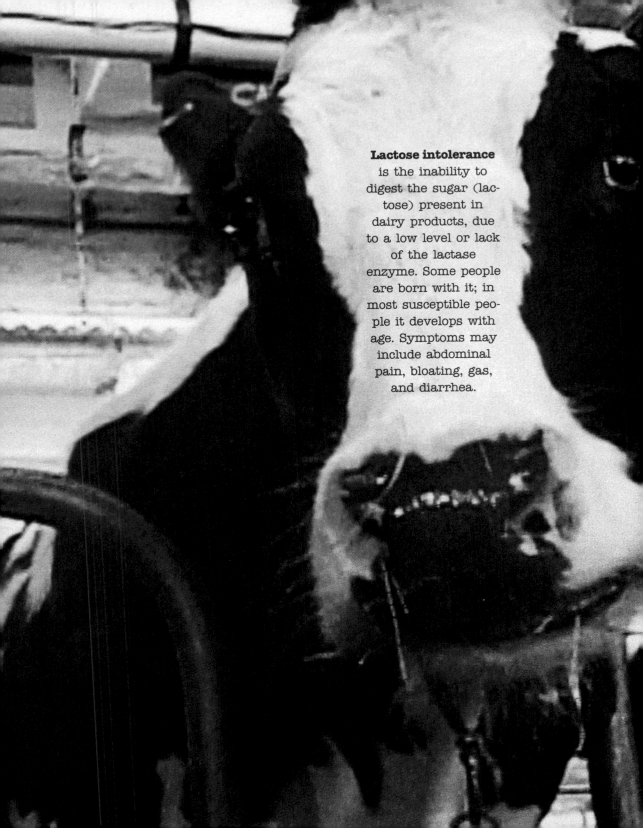

Lactose intolerance is the inability to digest the sugar (lactose) present in dairy products, due to a low level or lack of the lactase enzyme. Some people are born with it; in most susceptible people it develops with age. Symptoms may include abdominal pain, bloating, gas, and diarrhea.

**Recombinant
bovine growth
hormone (rBGH),**
a genetically engineered hormone that increases milk production,
has been permitted in U.S. dairy herds since
1985. rBGH-injected cows produce milk with
high levels of Insulin Growth Factor-1 (IGF-1);
recent research has found links between ele-
vated levels of IGF-1 and increased risk of
breast and prostate cancer. Since 1994,
every industrialized country in the world
except the United States (including Canada,
Japan, and all 15 nations of the European
Union) has banned rBGH milk. The United
Nations Food Standards Body refuses to
certify that rBGH is safe. According to the
Monsanto company, over a quarter of U.S.
milk cows are now in herds supplement-
ed with Posilac, its commercial version of
rBGH. Most of the country's dairy companies mix rBGH milk with non-rBGH
milk during processing; it's now in an
estimated 80–90 per cent of the U.S.
dairy supply.

Source: Ché Green. "Got rBGH?"
Independent Weekly, 7 August 2002.

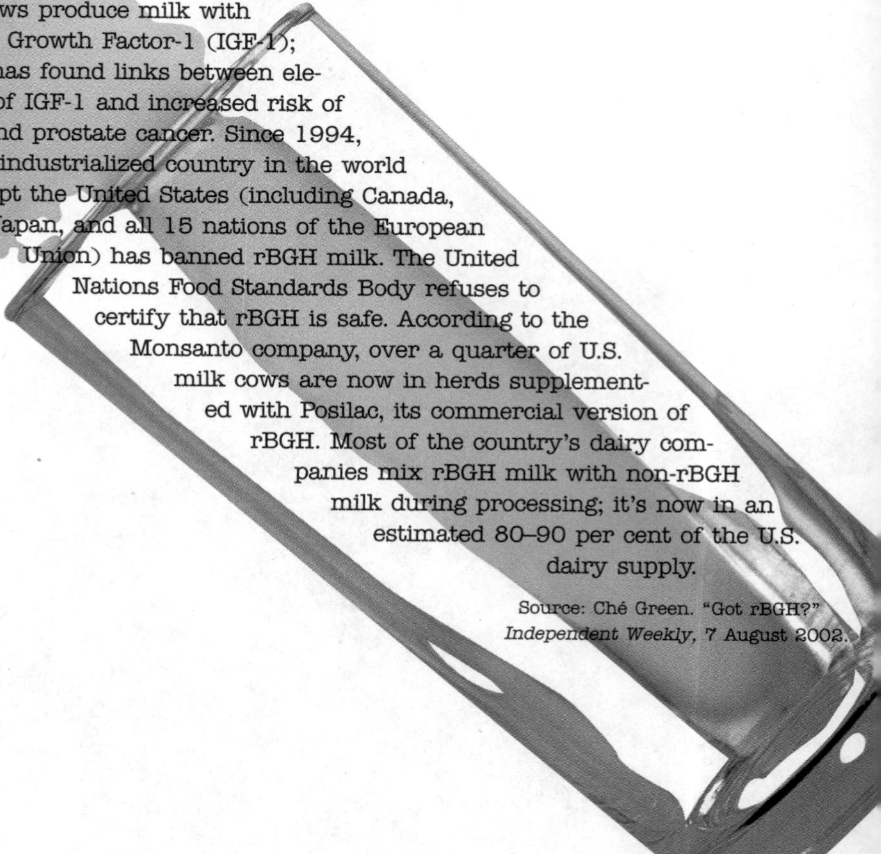

"You're lactose intolerant," she said.

I just looked at her with a confused expression on my face. As far as I knew, people who were lactose intolerant got sick to their stomach when they ate dairy, but I didn't have that problem. "I'm sorry?" I answered, wiping more snot away.

"You're lactose intolerant," she said again. "If you just cut dairy out of your diet, that runny nose will go away in a few days."

I just couldn't believe it. I told her about how I'd had the problem my whole life and about going to doctors and specialists to try and get rid of it, then this young girl takes one look at me and tells me all I have to do is cut out dairy?

"That's right," she said, "and your skin will clear up too."

It turned out that she had pretty much the same problem as me and was lucky enough to meet a health food nutritionist who diagnosed it as lactose intolerance. The nutritionist put her on a specialized diet that was dairy-free and she hadn't had the problem since. I found out later that we're all lactose intolerant; it's just that some people have worse reactions to dairy than others. That's probably got something to do with the fact that nature created cow's milk for baby cows, not humans. Milk does do a body good—a calf's body.

What the hell, I thought—after almost a quarter-century of snorting and coughing, I was about fed up with the whole mucus thing, so I decided to take the girl's advice just to see what would happen. I made an effort in the days following that bus ride to cut dairy right out of my diet— no milk, no cheese, no ice cream, no

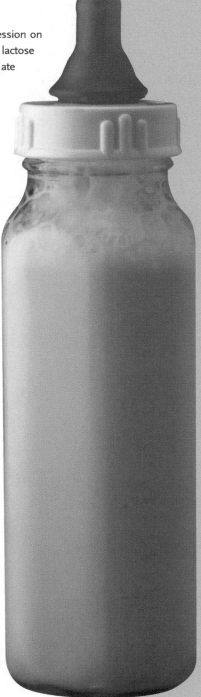

The U.S. Department of Agriculture's food guides promote consumption of dairy products as part of a healthy diet. The advisory committee for its Dietary Guidelines 2000 included people with affiliations to Dannon (maker of dairy products), the National Dairy Council, Nestlé (maker of ice creams and milk-based infant formula), and Slim-Fast (maker of milk-based diet products).

Source: Joanne Stepaniak. The Ultimate Uncheese Cookbook.

cream in coffee, and nothing with any dairy ingredients. Within a day I started to notice a difference. My runny nose was gone. My sinuses were clear for the first time in years, so my head stopped feeling like it was packed with cotton. I could hear better. I could breathe a lot easier, and my energy level and stamina increased. After about a week, my skin lost that red, blotchy look and the acne started clearing up. It was a total transformation.

I felt so fantastic within just a few days of cutting out dairy that it was easy for me to commit to never eating dairy again, and I've kept that promise to this day. I've been dosed a couple of times since then by ignorant waiters but knew right away because my body immediately showed flu symptoms. Other than that though, I've never looked back.

Quitting dairy cleared up my sinuses and my skin, but the whole experience did more than that: it was at that point that my whole way of thinking started to shift. If dairy had been having that much of an effect on my health and well-being, I thought, what the hell was eating at McDonald's and all the other negative shit I was doing having on me? For the first time in my life I started to feel this real need to acquire some degree of self-awareness about my diet and to start treating my body like the temple it should be. I finally woke up to the fact that there was a big gap between the life I was experiencing and the optimum life I could experience. I started to really think about what I was eating, to read books, talk to nutritionists, ask questions.

It shouldn't be that difficult to figure out, but it really is true that the more you look, the more you see. I went from not thinking twice about anything I put in my stomach to wanting to know absolutely everything I could about anything I ingested—where it came from, how it was produced, who produced it, and what effect the various ingredients and chemical components had on my body. I started to make connections, like

Raw Food Diet

Raw foodists eat only raw, uncooked, unheated, unprocessed organic food. Practitioners believe the food in this diet contains more enzymes because it is never heated over 116° Fahrenheit (47° Celsius). Because enzymes help break down food inside the body and are said to be the food's energy source, raw foodists strive to preserve the highest level of enzymes in their food possible. Raw foodists only eat certified organic foods because most commercially grown produce is sprayed with pesticides and other toxic substances that they believe are not good for the body. Although the terms are generally interchangeable, some raw foodists make a distinction between raw and "living" foods. Living foods are those in a "sprouted" state and are believed to have a higher enzyme activity than raw, unsprouted foods.

There are different types of raw foodists. Fruitarians only eat fruits, berries, and nuts. By doing this, they avoid killing the plant because they are only removing its fruit, leaving the living plant to bear fruit again. Even rarer categories of raw foodists include sproutarians, who only eat sprouts, and liquidarians, who only drink juice.

—KH.

Source: www.living-foods.com

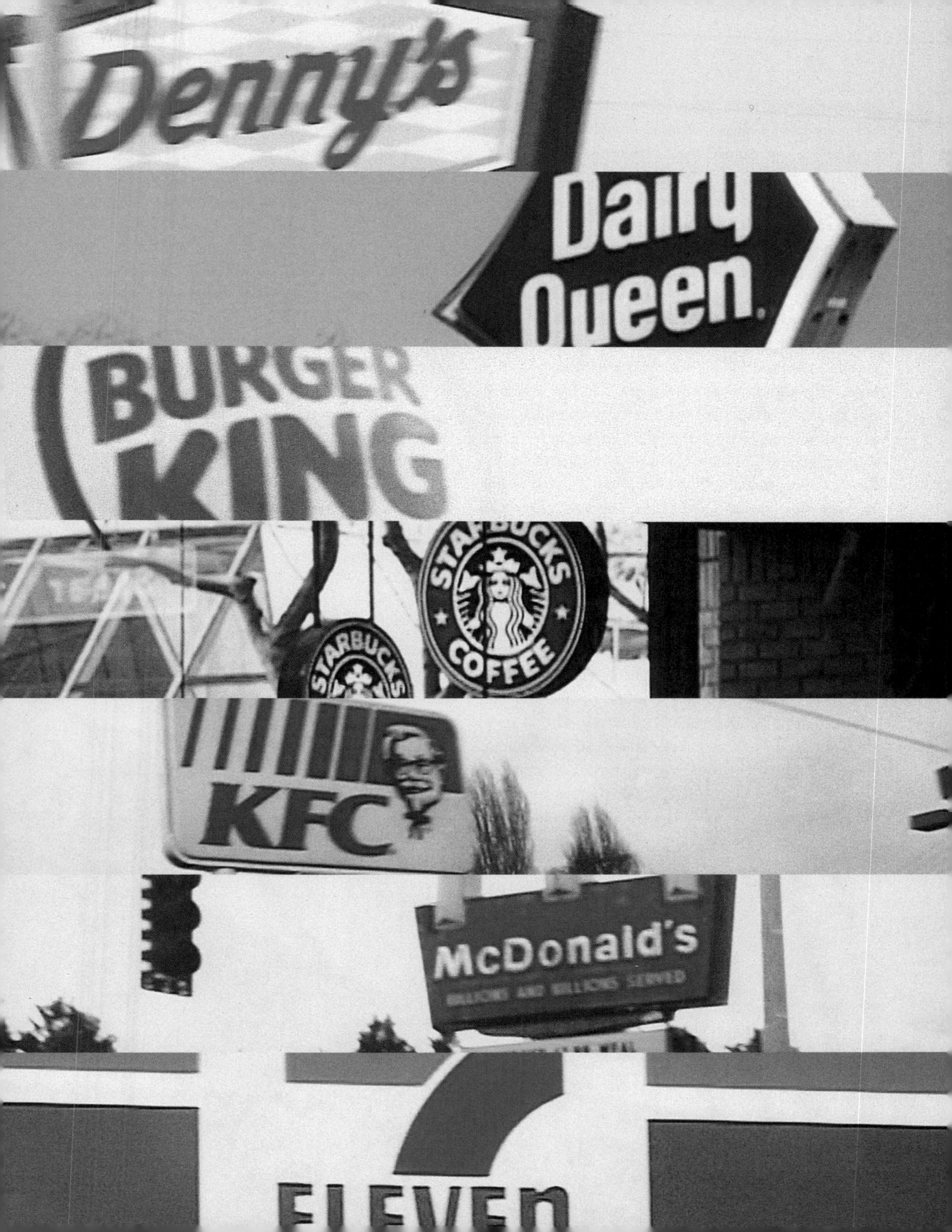
Denny's
Dairy Queen
BURGER KING
STARBUCKS COFFEE
STARBUCKS
KFC
McDonald's
ELEVEN

how every time I ate a burger all I wanted to do was just kick back and sit on the couch and watch TV, or maybe even take a nap. So my inspiration to become a vegan, someone who eats no animal products at all, really came from a desire to get more energy in my life, because eating dead animals was just zapping me.

Getting off meat wasn't an immediate change for me, like getting off dairy, but right around the same time I started to get into yoga, and I was meeting a lot of vegans. I was really inspired by talking with them and seeing how healthy and energetic they were. I kept at it, and eventually the combination of my changing diet and the yoga really started to pay dividends. Just like my nose and skin cleared up after I dumped dairy, I noticed my energy level went through the roof. I found I didn't need to sleep as much at night and I never felt like napping during the day anymore. On top of that, the yoga made me way more flexible, and that translated into more speed and quickness on the basketball court, which was a little unexpected bonus.

When I started to see my body change and felt the shift happening in my overall health, I knew there was no going back. Then when my kids came along I started a whole new shift, a mental one, away from the self-centered focus of my past to a new awareness of other people and the whole planet. It was around that time that I really started to think about how my life choices were affecting other people and the environment. I decided that I wanted to do what

I could to make a bigger change happen. That's when I started to get it—personal transformation equals planetary transformation.

The more research I did, the more I saw how people today, especially in the United States, are digging their own grave with their fork, and not just because of what their diet is doing to them personally. After making the switch to a vegan diet, I wanted to take the next step, so I started to learn more and more about organic alternatives, which shifted me a little further down my evolutionary path. The information is out there—about pesticides and herbicides, genetically modified food, hormone and steroid injections in beef cattle and dairy cows, factory farming. But most people trust what they're told—meat makes you strong, milk does a body good.

Well, once my eyes were finally opened, I couldn't believe the shit I started to see. I walked down the snack aisle at the 7-11, for a long time one of my favorite places to eat, and looked at all the candy bars, Doritos, Funions, and suddenly I realized that there was basically not one thing in the whole fucking store that I would eat anymore. I picked up a package of M&Ms and read the ingredients for the first time: red dye #5, red dye #4, artificial flavor, artificial color, methylparabin, petroleum products. Petroleum products, I thought, what the hell is that? What the hell is any of that shit? I ate crap like that for years and it wasn't even food. This should be obvious but if you can't pronounce it and Mother Nature didn't make it, it probably shouldn't be in your body.

Taking off my corporate feed bag also opened my eyes up to the way our society is bombarded constantly with food propaganda that is at best misleading and at worst a downright lie. Think about it: McDonald's uses little plastic toys and a clown to bribe little kids to eat factory meat and french fries boiled in partially hydrogenated oil. They call them "Happy Meals." Happy for who? Not the cows, and not the kids either if they keep eating that crap. My friends' daughter died at age twenty-three of leukemia. But I believe she died of fast food—it's all she ever ate. You turn on the TV and you've got John Elway with a white moustache on his lip asking you if you've "Got Milk?" as if there's something wrong with you if you don't. Then we've got Coke telling us it's the "Real Thing." Have you ever read the ingredients in a can of Coke? There's nothing real about it.

When I look back on my former life now, having

gone through my food detox and made the difficult transition to a plant-based, organic diet, I just can't believe the way I ate for almost thirty years. Worse than that, I can't believe the way I let myself be lied to about what I was eating for almost thirty years. It's like I was in a trance, not asking any questions about anything. If it tasted good, I ate it. Hell, John Elway says it's OK. And the vast majority of people are like that—more interested in food that "comforts" them than food that nourishes them. That's especially true in the United States, and the proof is in the fact that the U.S. is among the most obese nations in the world. There are many substances for people to anesthetize themselves, like booze or drugs, but I believe highly processed corporate food is the number one drug. And what a withdrawal when you quit!

An amazing thing happens when you start to wean yourself off the corporate boob. Once you drop the dairy, the fat, and the refined sugar, and all the chemical and biological additives that come with them, you begin to shed what I call your "false body." When you eat food that is highly processed or has biochemicals in it that your system doesn't recognize, your body does one of two things: it eliminates them if it can or it stores them if it can't. On top of that, if your body doesn't get enough nutritional value from the food you eat, it stays in a perpetual state of semi-starvation, constantly trying to store up nutrients as fat whenever it can because it can't be sure you'll give it what it needs tomorrow and the next day. After years and years of storing up fat and other crap you can't use, your body ends up with a layer of "extraness," a false body that surrounds the hard, lean, healthy, essential body nature gave you. Most people lug around a false body, and some are bigger than others. Some people even attach a layer of emotional flab to the physical one to insulate themselves from the world even more. I have a number of friends in this situation. I'm no stranger to insulating myself from pain, but why go into that now? Do as I say, not as I do.

Once you start feeding your body though, instead of just filling it, your false body loses its reason to be. First of all, because you're no longer taking in all kinds of stuff you don't need and can't use, your body doesn't

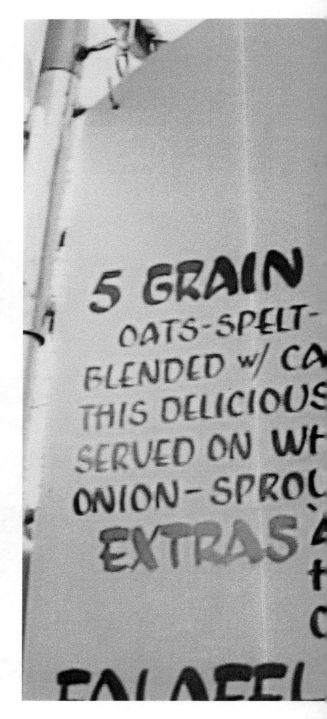

EMP BURGER- 5 50

LLET-HEMP SEEDS & QUINOA ARE
OTS, LEGUMES & SPICES TO MAKE
URGER. FORTIFIED w/ 'HEMP NUT'
E GRAIN BUN w/ LETTUCE-TOMATO
- KETCHUP & MUSTARD.
S' HOMEMADE 1000 ISLAND
MP NUT SAUCE .50 AVOCADO .T
ESE .75 (O.G. CHEDDAR OR NON-DAIRY
5 50 'ALS' ONE OF A KIND

What is Vegetarianism?

Vegetarianism means different things to different people. Some people believe the only true vegetarian is someone who eats no animal products at all. Others will call someone who only avoids eating a certain kind of meat a vegetarian. Bearing this in mind, there are many different types of vegetarianism, each with its own philosophy and restrictions.

Although vegetarianism has been central to a number of cultures for millennia, its practice has been inconsistent for the most part throughout history. The first well-known vegetarian was the Greek mathematician Pythagoras, who popularized the practice throughout ancient Greece. Vegetarianism was also a central tenet of the Manichean religion, which began in Persia in the third century and eventually spread to Europe and China. Before converting to Catholicism, St. Augustine was a Manichean.

The practice of vegetarianism has always existed on the fringes of Western society, but that appears to be changing. In the 1800s, the Vegetarian Society in the United Kingdom had a membership of only about a few thousnd people, but more than twelve million North Americans classified themselves as vegetarians in 1994, and their numbers continue to rise today.

Most people subscribe to a diet that is called "instinctive eating." They choose foods based upon what their senses find appetizing. In other words, they eat what they feel like, and do so instinctively. The instinctive diet includes a variety of meats, grains, dairy, vegetables, and fruit, and makes no distinction between natural and processed foods. Vegetarians, however, make a conscious effort to break away from instinctive eating patterns based on taste alone.

The most common form of vegetarianism is known as lacto-ovo. A lacto-ovo vegetarian does not eat meat in any form (this includes fish, red meat, or fowl), but does eat dairy (lacto) and eggs (ovo). Lacto vegetarians eat no meat or eggs, but do drink milk. Ovo vegetarians do not drink milk or eat meat, but do eat eggs.

There are many individuals who consider themselves "semi-vegetarians." For example, a person who does not eat red meat but does consume fish and fowl might consider themselves semi-vegetarian. In fact, these individuals are often called pesco-pollo vegetarians. Likewise, those who eat fowl (chicken, duck, turkey, etc.) but don't eat red meat are called pollo-vegetarians; and those who eat fish and seafood but don't eat red meat or fowl are called pesco-vegetarians.

But these diets are not recognized as "true" vegetarian diets by the Vegetarian Society, formed in England in 1847.

Veganism

Partly in reaction to the rather ambiguous meaning of "vegetarian," the Vegan Society was formed in Great Britain in 1944. A vegan is someone who eats no animal-derived foods—no meat, poulty, fish, dairy, eggs, or honey. As well as health and environmental concerns, the basis for veganism is respect for all animal life. Therefore, many vegans also avoid using products derived from animals, such as fur, leather, and wool. They also avoid products tested on animals, such as some cosmetics and household products.

—KH.

Sources: The Vegetarian Society of the United Kingdom (www.vegsoc.org); The Vegan Society (www.vegansociety.com).

need to find a place to store the excess crap until it can get rid of it. Then, if you're only taking in wholesome, nutritious, organic food, your body will find a way to utilize every bit of it, like the highly efficient survival engine it's supposed to be. And once your body feels it can trust you to keep that wholesome, nutritious organic food coming on a daily basis, it can stop storing nutrients as fat in an effort to keep your sorry ass alive. Pretty soon you'll see a whole new person emerging.

Something else I've learned is that when you eat food that doesn't actually feed your body, you spend a lot more time eating and a lot more time feeling hungry. This is because most people get so little energy and nutrition from the food they eat that their body has to keep calling constantly for the essential nutrients it needs to keep the engine running. So if you just ate the Double Combo burger with the Biggy fries and the Super Size soda and an hour or so later your brain is telling you you're still hungry, what it's really saying is, "Hey stupid, give me something I can use."

Since I've been eating a totally organic, plant-based diet, I find that I really don't need to eat that much at all to keep my energy level right up there. Some days I might be working from 6:00 in the morning until 9:00 at night, doing something really physical in some hot location, and I find I survive just fine munching on fruit and raw vegetables all day. My diet supports me energetically. In fact, more than anything, the changes in my diet came from a desire to optimize my energy level. I can fly from Hawaii to Europe, halfway around the world, and just get off the plane and keep right on going. I don't get jet lag. I don't seem to have a problem with time differences, and I travel quite a lot. I find my mental clarity is a lot better after I eat a huge organic salad than it ever was after I ate a burger—that's if I could stay awake. In fact, in every way I feel like I'm performing at a higher efficiency level, a higher level of consciousness, and that's what it's all about. By cleansing my body of the stuff that didn't

need to be there, I opened my vessel up to receiving more energy, more awareness, more emotion.

Today I feel like food plays the role in my life that it's supposed to play: it is the healer that makes it possible for me to experience my life, rather than the comforter that allows me to sleepwalk through it. It wasn't easy getting to this point though; I had to train my body to crave things that were good for it, instead of things I was conditioned to believe tasted good. That takes discipline and practice. There were lots of times along the way when my brain would latch on to things that reminded it of the comfort food diet I ate in the past, like the smell of freshly baked cookies or muffins, and some part of my body would just go, "I have to have that." There have even been times along the way when I broke down and ate stuff that I know now is not for human consumption, like glazed doughnuts, but almost right away my body protested. See, once your body sheds that outer layer and gets a taste for that good, nutritious organic food, it can't take the processed shit anymore. Even one doughnut feels like a whole loaf of bread in your gut.

It takes a little longer for your brain to catch on, though. There needs to be a mental shift there before you start to understand that all those great smells you get from baked, fried, roasted, or barbequed food are really the smell of most of the good stuff being cooked right out of it, if there was any good stuff in it in the first place. Eventually, you come to the realization that there's a sort of law of diminishing returns with all that comfort food you used to crave so much. Sure it smells good, and your mouth might want it, but the rest of your body sure doesn't. As soon as you get that, you'll find yourself dreaming about the smell of fresh fruit and salivating over the thought of eating a big, fresh organic salad.

One of the best things about getting off the corporate food and going organic is that it opens up a whole new world of food to you. When your brain is tuned in, you'll find that you start to notice cool vegetarian restau-

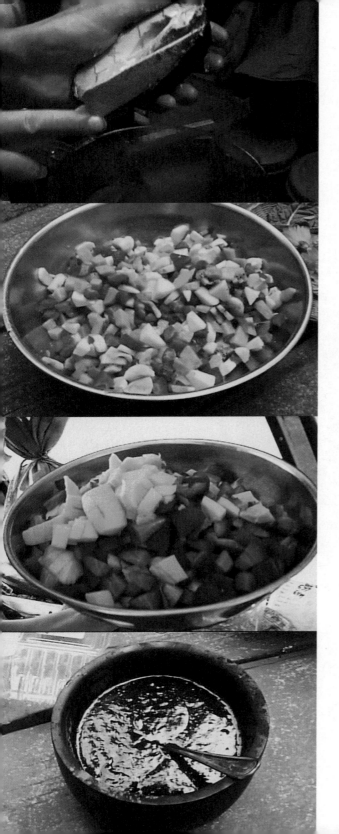

rants that you didn't even know were there before. A lot of people worry that they'll lose "variety" in their diet if they go vegetarian or vegan, but there's a lot of great vegetarian cookbooks out there that can give you all the variety you'll ever need. Besides, there are cultures in the world that adhere to a strictly vegetarian diet for religious reasons, and they've been managing pretty well for literally thousands of years. There really is a whole different world out there if you want to find it; you just have to be willing to get off that narrow road that most people choose to travel.

With just a little effort, it's not hard to find great sources of organic food. There are some mainstream grocery stores out there that make the effort to carry organic fruit and vegetables, and sometimes even organically raised, grass-fed beef if you're still struggling with that. But if you can't get organic where you usually buy your food, drop into the health food store you've been passing by for years and ask for help. Better yet, get up early some Saturday morning and take a trip to your local farmer's market—most big cities have at least one—and talk to the organic farmers. There are even some growers' co-operatives out there that will put together a box of organic produce for you and deliver it to your house once a week, and there's nothing difficult about that.

So you say you want to change the world? Well, I say that's great; go change it, and you can start today by changing your diet. I know because I did it. I may be a skinny, raw food–eating yoga freak today, but I come from the same super-sized world as everybody else. I learned that you can create a life free of poison and genetic manipulation, and expose yourself to just those things that we know are good for us: earth, air, water, and sunlight. I also learned that you can stop pouring money into the pockets of corporations that don't treat your Mother right. And if you don't think you're ready to make a big change in your life, then even a small shift in the right direction will make a difference.

Personal transformation equals planetary transformation—if I can do it, anybody can do it.

Get on the bus.

Organic foods

The definition and labelling of "organic food" is a contentious issue. In October 2002, the U.S. Department of Agriculture's (USDA) National Organic Program was created to set organic food standards. In the United States, food labelled "organic" must be produced according to strict legal criteria.

- The producer must use methods and materials that do not harm the environment.

- Crops are rotated from field to field, rather than growing the same crop year after year. Cover crops such as clover are planted to add nutrients to the soil and prevent weeds.

- The land on which organic food is grown has been free of known and perceived toxic and persistent chemical pesticides and fertilizers for three years prior to certification.

- Use of genetically modified organisms is not permitted.

- Minimal processing is used, with no artificial ingredients, preservatives, or irradiation.

- Organic meat, poultry, and egg products come from farms that have been inspected and where rigorous standards have been met, such as using organic feed, not using antibiotics or hormones, and giving animals access to outdoors, fresh air, and sunlight. Market animals are raised without the use of toxic, persistent pesticides, antibiotics, and parasiticides.

- Production methods must meet all federal, state, and local health regulations; work in harmony with the environment; build biological diversity; and foster healthy soil and growing conditions.

- Detailed records of methods and materials used in growing or processing organic products must be maintained and audited. All methods and materials must be annually inspected by a third party certifier approved by the USDA. All farmers and handlers must maintain and regularly update written organic plans detailing their management practices.

- In order to bear the USDA "Certified Organic" seal, a product must contain 95 to 100 per cent organic ingredients.

Sources: Sustainable Table; USDA Agricultural Marketing Service. "The National Organic Program: Labeling and Marketing Information," USDA, October 2002.

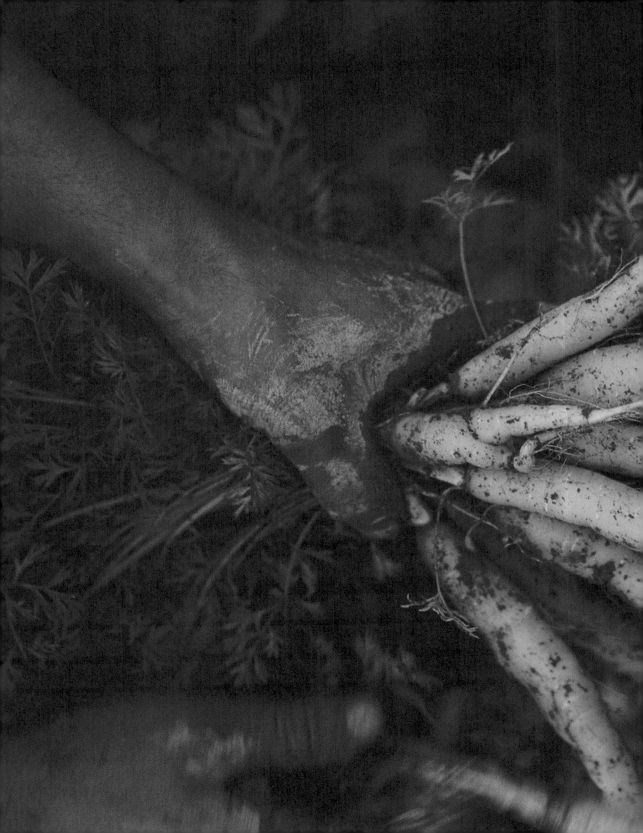

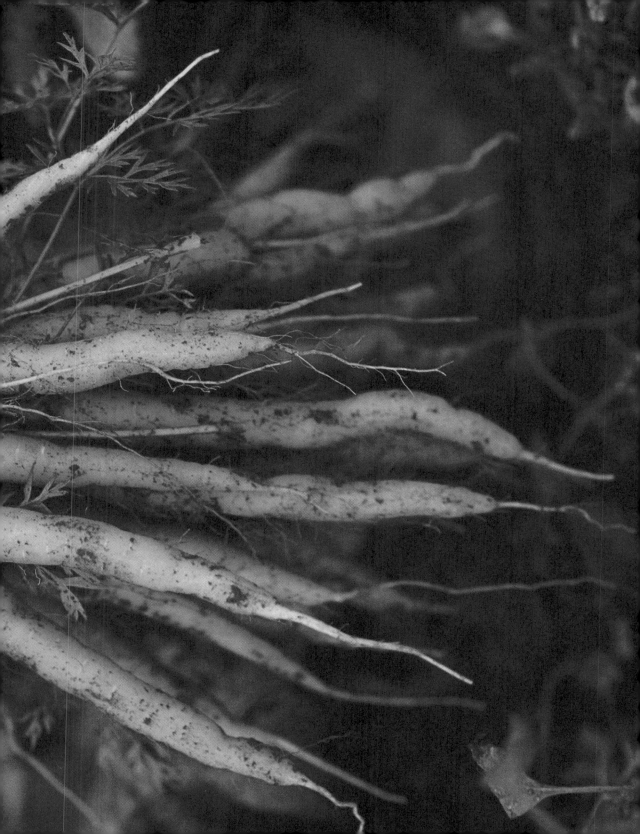

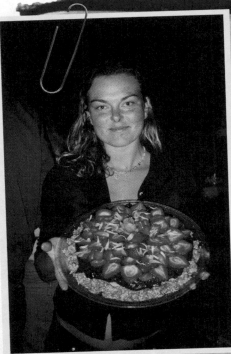

Chocolate of the Gods Mousse

THIS "CHOCOLATE OF THE GODS MOUSSE" CAME TO ME IN A DREAM. (LITERALLY). THE SECRET IS AVOCADO FOR A SUMPTUOUS, CREAMY BASE! A TRULY DECADENT CHOCOLATE TO SATISFY ANY SENSUAL SWEET TOOTH. RAW CAROB POWDER CAN BE USED AS A BASE WITH THE COMPLEMENT OF A GOOD ORGANIC COCOA TO LIFT THE FLAVOR TO DIVINITY (I RECOMMEND GREEN & BLACK COCOA POWDER— FOR THE INTEGRITY OF THE COMPANY AND THEIR ASSURANCE THAT THE COCOA IS TREATED WITH THE RESPECT OF LOW TEMPERATURES TO PROTECT LUSCIOUS FLAVOR AND QUALITY).

THIS MOUSSE CAN BE PREPARED AS A PARFAIT, LAYERED WITH BERRIES IN A WINE OR MARTINI GLASS FOR A STUNNING APPEARANCE. OR THE MOUSSE CAN BE COMPLEMENT-ED BY A CRUMBLY NUT CRUST TO SERVE AS A PIE. DEFINITELY TOP WITH FRESH MINT LEAVES, AND LICK THE BOWL.

WITH WELL SEASONED LOVE,
Renée

INGREDIENTS (*Yields 1 dish*)

- 3 avocados
- 1/2-cup maple syrup, or 1-1/4 cup soft dates (as an alternative sweetener)
- 2 to 4 tablespoons organic evaporated cane juice* (optional—for a sweeter tooth)
- 1 tablespoon non-alcoholvanilla extract
- 1-1/2 tablespoon cold-pressed coconut butter or olive oil (I recommend Omega Nutrition coconut butter as it does not smell or taste like coconut, which interferes with the fine flavor of chocolate)
- 3/4-cup raw carob powder
- 4 tablespoons organic cocoa powder (add a touch more for "darker" chocolate—I adore dark chocolate) If raw carob is not available, use a total of 2/3-cup cocoa (as cocoa has a much stronger flavor than carob), adding more to taste
- 1 pint raspberries or sliced strawberries
- Fresh mint leaves

*An unrefined, organic "raw sugar" produced by a company called Wholesome Foods; available in most health food and natural food stores.

TECHNIQUE

- If you are using dates: Pit the dates and cover with fresh water to soften for 5 to 15 minutes.
- In a food processor: Blend avocados (scooped out of the skin without the pit!), with sweet ingredients, vanilla and coconut butter or olive oil until smooth.
- Spoon in carob and cocoa powder and blend until creamy.
- Layer with fresh berries in a wine or martini glass and top with fresh mint leaves.
- This mousse will stay fresh in a sealed container in the fridge for 3-4 days.

CRUMBLE CRUST

- 1/2-cup almonds, soaked in fresh water for 8 hours
- 3/4-cup pecans
- 3/4-cup walnuts
- 4 to 6 soft dates, pitted
- 2 tablespoons maple syrup or raw honey
- 2 teaspoons cinnamon
- pinch sundried sea salt

TECHNIQUE

- In a food processor: Chop nuts into a fine meal.
- Add dates and maple or honey and chop until well mixed.
- Add cinnamon and a pinch of salt.
- The texture should be crumbly and sticky.
- Press evenly into a pie plate.
- Sliced strawberries or bananas can be layered into the bottom of the pie crust.
- Spread the Chocolate of the Gods Mousse evenly into the pie crust and generously top with fresh berries and mint.

Source: Renée Loux Underkoffler, "Da Kine Kitchen" recipes at Voice Yourself (http://www.voiceyourself.com/09_dakinekitchen/09_easy.php#12). Look here for more raw food recipes by Renée.

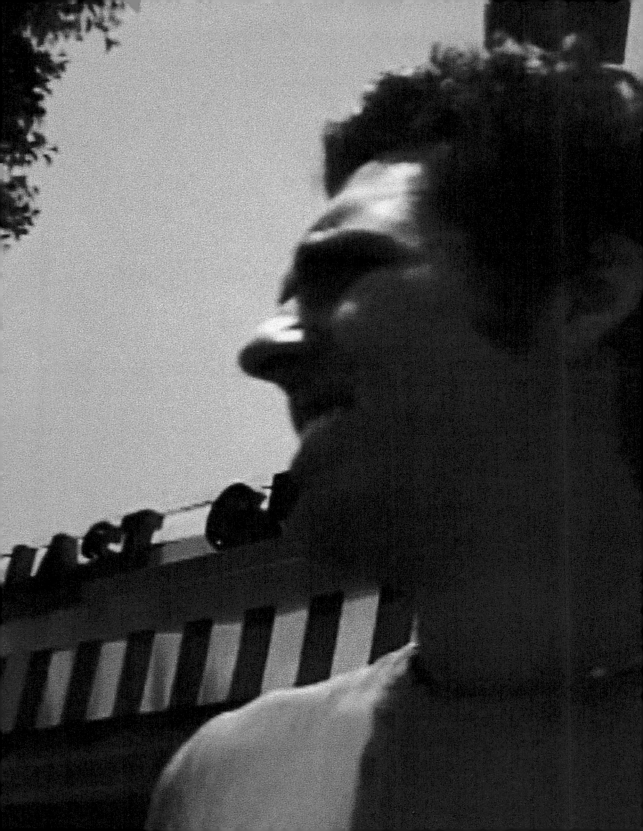

JEDI'S JOURNEY

Steve "Jedi" Clark

I was born in a place called Lynchburg, Virginia. It's a small town in a rural area about 175 miles southwest of Washington, D.C. If you ever saw *Dukes of Hazzard*, you can kind of get an image in your head of the place I grew up—there were a lot of farmers, a lot of hunters, and a lot of rednecks. Not a single hippie though, that I remember anyway.

When I was still little my mom moved us to a really small town, called Goode, Virginia, which is about eight miles from Lynchburg, into a farmhouse with about a hundred acres and a bunch of cows, and that was basically where I spent my childhood. It was a cool place to be a kid, that's for sure; for me, growing up in rural

Virginia was all about building forts in the woods and hangin' out by the railway tracks.

We left Virginia when I was about thirteen and headed south. I'd have to say we knocked around a fair bit, and I guess that's why I'm kind of a restless soul today. I even managed to make a few stops in three or four trailer parks along the way. I went to high school in Goose Creek, South Carolina, although most of the people I went to school with, and the teachers especially, probably wouldn't have known I was even there. I was lazy and kind of a gawky kid, so I tended to hang around with the outsiders. I did play Junior Varsity basketball one year and JV football another year, though. Then I asked myself why I was willing to take so much physical abuse and just said, "To hell with this." After that I discovered pot, became a stoner, and figured I'd found my calling in life.

After high school, we moved to Orlando, Florida, and it was about that time, fresh out of high school and motivated to do just about nothing, that I decided it was time for me to leave the nest and "find myself." So, like any self-respecting slacker, I hooked up with some guys at a Grateful Dead concert, hopped in their camper, and headed out to the West Coast. It took us a couple of months to get there; we just followed the Dead from place to place until we made it to California, and that's where I got out.

I don't know if it was the sun or the ocean or the pot but in Lotusland the gypsy in me just took over. I lived a real alternative existence, making T-shirts and going to Grateful Dead concerts, burning weed and traveling around on my thumb. I spent time in San Francisco, San Diego, Yosemite, and Lake Tahoe; sometimes I had a place to live, sometimes I didn't. I was just kind of a lost soul, or a free spirit, depending on how you look at it. But I didn't care. I was lovin' life and I was happy just to float along on the breeze.

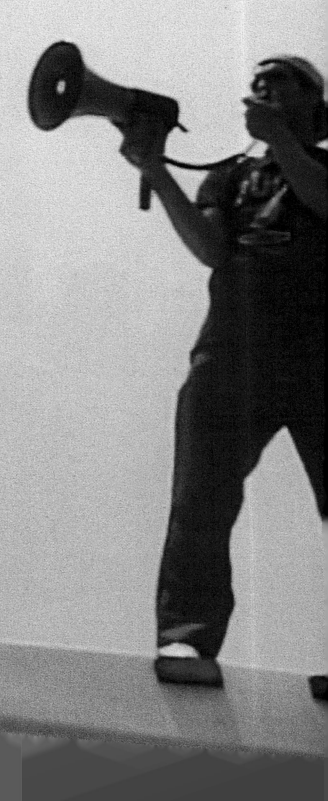

Things changed for me in 1996. That's when an uncle of mine who happens to be an actor landed a role in a television show. He said he could get me a job working around the studio, so I moved to Hollywood and actually got myself an apartment. I started as basically a gofer on a show called *Boston Common*, which a few people might remember, although it wasn't on for very long. For the first time in my life I had a job and an apartment and it felt pretty weird. I was actually stable.

I thought to myself, "Man, here you are, the stoner from Lynchburg, livin' in Hollywood, working in the entertainment industry—how great is that?"

It was pretty cool—I was getting to hang out with the beautiful people, I was getting fed every day for free, I was getting free long distance phone calls—I'd pretty much hit the slacker jackpot, you could say.

Then, of course, it all blew up on me. *Boston Common* got cancelled after one season and I was out of a job again. Luckily though, I managed to make friends with the guys who created the show and they had started working on a new one that was going to be called, believe it or not, *Will & Grace*. It was cool because I kind of saw *Will & Grace* come together from the ground up. I watched my friends writing it and having all these meetings with the network about how it was going to be a show, then it wasn't going to be a show, then it was. Then it got picked up and—poof—I had a job again.

So *Will & Grace* became a huge hit and my perfect pot-smoking, beach-sittin', Hollywood slacker life was back on track. I found out pretty fast that working on a hit show is a lot more fun than working on one that's headed for cancellation. The mood on the set is always up and you get to meet lots of famous guest stars. I became really friendly with one of the producers, Jimmy Burrows, who was one of the main guys behind shows like *Cheers*, *Taxi*, *Friends*, and *Frasier*.

So I worked on *Will & Grace* for a few months, doing my coffee thing, and then for this one particular episode we all had to fly out to New York to shoot, which was another cool first-time freebie for me. When we were in New York, there was this big cast party and there were all kinds of celebrities there. I was just basically hanging around the shrimp bowl, trying to look like I hadn't just wandered in off the street when Jimmy Burrows came up to me and said, "Hey man, there's someone here I'd like you to meet, you guys are going to love each other." He disappeared into the crowd and after a few minutes he comes back with Woody Harrelson behind him.

Now, meeting Woody was a really awesome experience for me, which was weird because I'd been working in Hollywood for a while by then and I'd been around plenty of celebrities and they didn't really impress me that much. The truth is I never really got caught up in the whole Hollywood thing. But Woody was different, I guess because

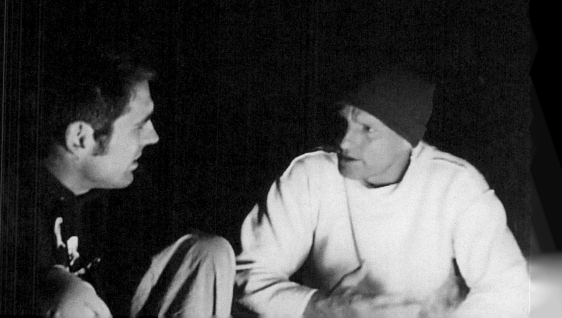

I knew he was pro pot, or at least pro hemp, although at that time I didn't know you could make anything out of weed other than a joint. But he seemed to be on the same wavelength as me on a lot of levels and I looked at him as a fellow burner who just happened to be a famous actor.

Well, Jimmy was right—Woody and I really did hit it off. After Jim introduced us, we stood in the corner shooting the shit for about an hour about all kinds of things we had in common—growing up poor in a small town, different kinds of music, movies, whatever. Finally Woody decided he better move around and talk to some

Woody showed up for rehearsals and he remembered me from the party in New York and we just kind of struck up our conversation again like we had been together just the day before. He worked on the show for a few weeks and over that time we bonded and became sort of buddies on the set.

I think Woody first spoke to me about the SOL Tour in October or November 2000. Of course, it wasn't the "SOL Tour" then, it was just a bike trip that he was planning to take down the coast with his brothers. For months I listened to Woody talking about this trip and all

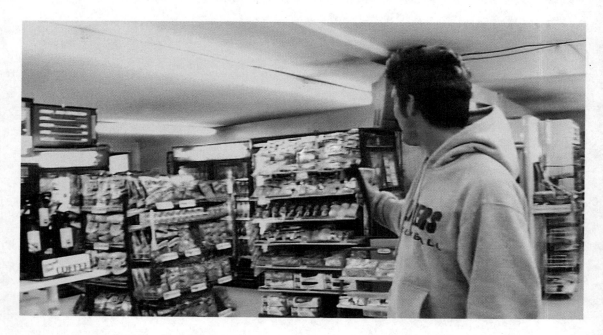

other people and we shook hands and I thought that was it. It was cool though, because just before he left he came back over to me and made a point of saying he was glad we met and that we should hook up again when we were both back in L.A. Of course I said that would be cool, but I didn't think it would ever happen.

Then, about three or four months later, I showed up for work one day back in Hollywood on the set of *Will & Grace* and Jimmy Burrows came up to me and said, "Hey man, guess what? Your buddy Woody Harrelson is guesting on the show."

the shit they were planning to do. As the time for the trip approached, it started to get bigger and all these other people started to get involved. Then Woody told me they were going to live in a biofuel-powered bus called the Mothership and stop to give lectures on the environment along the way. Suddenly his little bike trip had turned into this whole activist crusade, and I started thinking to myself, "Man, I've got to get in on this thing."

By the time April 2001 arrived, I was good buddies with Woody and all but I didn't really feel like I knew him well enough to just say, "Hey Woody, man, put me on the bus," because the people involved were all his family and his really close friends. On the other hand, it was killing me knowing that this really cool thing was going to happen and I was so close to being a part of it. So I just kind of hung around, helping any way I could and smiling a lot. Right up until the last minute it didn't look like it was going to happen for me. Then, just about two hours before the bus was going to leave L.A. to drive up to meet everybody in Seattle, Woody called me up and said, "Hey man, we want you to come along on the bus just to kind of help out with the bikes and stuff."

was really kind of magical the way it all came together for me, and I can't remember ever feeling so free.

So I was on the SOL Tour, and that was cool just from a fun perspective, but I had no idea how the experience would affect my life in a larger sense. I mean, I knew Woody and his brothers and friends were going to ride bikes back down the coast and live in the bus; and I knew that they planned to make stops along the way to talk to people about the environment and eating right and other stuff that Woody is very passionate about. So I knew it was a good cause and the whole thing had a

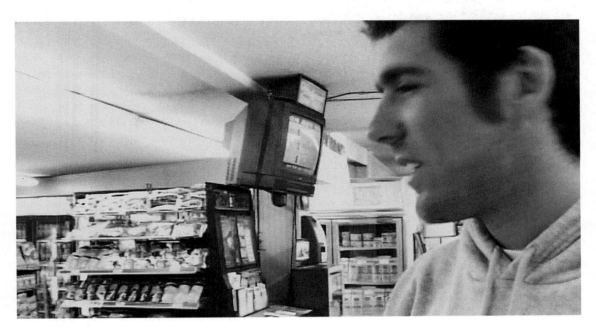

I was so happy, I think I almost screamed when he said it. Then I freaked out because I only had a couple of hours to pack and get my shit together and find someone to take care of my dogs, but somehow it all came together. I filled a knapsack, got a ride to where the bus was and jumped in. It was probably the most amazing moment of my life—one minute I was bummed because I knew this great thing was happening and I was sitting at home, and the next minute I was sitting on this cool organic bus heading up the coast to Seattle—just me, the mechanic, and the bus driver. It

great energy about it, but I sure didn't think that that energy would have an effect on me.

Come to think of it, there were a lot of things I didn't know about when I jumped on that biofuel-powered bus and headed off with Woody's tribe. I didn't know who I was going to be living on top of for days on end, for one thing. I mean, when I got on that bus I met my first yoga instructor, my first vegan chef, my first hemp activist, my first environmental activist lawyer. All I could say was, "Hey, I'm Steve; I'm a Deadhead production assistant from Virginia."

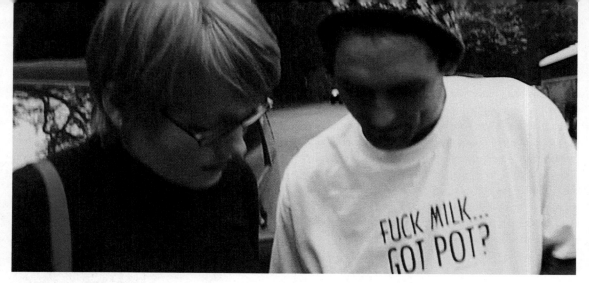

I also didn't know that they were all going to be eating nothing but raw food for the whole trip. I had no idea about that until I showed up in Seattle and hooked up with Woody and the rest of them. I knew Woody was a freak about his diet just from hanging out with him, but I had no idea he was a hardcore raw-foodist.

Now nobody made me sign anything before I got on the bus promising to eat raw food myself or anything like that, but when Woody told me that that's what everybody else was going to be doing, I figured I owed it to him for bringing me along to at least try it. Anyway, it would've been pretty rude of me to be living on their bus and walking around drinking a Big Gulp out of a Styrofoam cup and eating hoagies all the time. Just as they were loading up the bus, I spotted a Burger King across the street and I thought to myself, "Man, this is lookin' pretty granola; this may be it for meat for a while. I don't know the next time I'll be able to eat some meat and I don't even know the next time I'll be near a store where I can get a candy bar or something."

So I walked across the street to Burger King and ordered three Whoppers and just wolfed 'em all down. It was April 10, 2001, and it was the last time I ate beef.

The amazing thing was, once I got on the bus and we got going, Renée, the raw food chef, started making up these fantastic veggie meals and after a while I found that I didn't even desire that old shit—at least most of the time. You have to remember, I grew up eating fried baloney, white bread, gallons of milk, Lucky Charms, and Cocoa Crispies. But that was all I knew; I thought I was

eating good. In fact, like lots of people, I always figured food was food, and I believed that right up until I got on that bus. Maybe my mom thought she knew something about nutrition, but I don't think she really knew. She thought she was doing the right things by her kids. I mean, that's what everybody eats in the South: meatloaf, mashed potatoes, and meat, meat, meat, meat.

And as far as learning about nutrition in school goes, you can forget that. I do remember something about there being four basic food groups, but I think that was maybe a one-day class. The teacher got up and said, "OK, eat vegetables." And we all said, "Yeah, OK," and that was it.

In rural Virginia when I was growing up, you had to search for that kind of information, because they sure didn't teach it to you in school. Even to this day, if you say you're a vegetarian I bet they don't even know what that is in places like where I come from. In fact, you'd probably get beat up if you said you were a vegetarian; it'd be like saying you're a Communist.

Now I'm not going to sit here and try to tell you that I didn't have any trouble with the whole raw food thing; it would probably be impossible for any normal person not to. More than a couple of times, I let it slide and sneaked out to find a local mini market to stock up on a couple of bottles of soda and maybe a few Snickers bars, so I was getting my junk food fix now and again at the beginning. But those cravings got less and less as the trip wore on and I began to feel better and better physically.

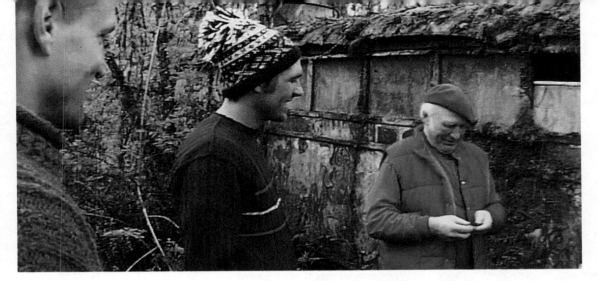

I guess it was only human to have those cravings. If you've been eating that way your whole life, your body thinks it needs that can of Coke, and it needs that Snickers bar, but it doesn't. I found out there's a lot of things your body thinks it needs that it doesn't need at all.

I remember one time, after I had sneaked out at night to buy candy bars, I felt so dirty being around the people on the bus and pretending to be as raw as them. I went up to Woody and said, "Hey dude, I feel really shitty about it, but I'm on the chocolate man. I just can't seem to get off it." I felt so bad, like a little kid going to the teacher to admit he'd done something terrible.

Woody just laughed at me and said, "It's OK brother, you're an addict. You're addicted to refined sugar, but you can beat it man. Keep fighting."

When I thought about it, I knew he was right. I'd spent three decades getting hooked on that white shit, so it was going to take a little while to get off it. But the fact is, the craving is all in your head; you don't really need the meat, or the chocolate, or the dairy, it's just that in your mind you miss it.

So I kept at it. Other than the bad shit I was sneaking at night, I was eating all the raw stuff everyone else was eating. Of course, I probably couldn't have done it at all if I hadn't had a great raw food chef on board. I was just amazed at all the things Renée could do to make the raw food tastier and more interesting. She made this one dish called Chocolate Avocado Pie that was totally raw and organic but tasted just like a Hershey's Kiss Jell-O Pudding Pop or something. It was incredible. But any-body can do it, and all you've got to do is put a little effort into learning how.

When people think raw, they tend to think of raw carrots or raw broccoli, something that a rabbit would eat, and yeah, that does seem boring. But the raw food I shared with Woody and his friends on the SOL Tour was nothing like that. And it's true: it does make you feel great. What they were telling me all throughout the Tour makes perfect sense to me now: if you eat food that's alive, you're going to feel alive; and if you eat food that's dead, you're going to feel dead. It's pretty basic.

I can honestly say I didn't join the SOL Tour to change my life or to make some kind of statement about the world or how people should live. For me, it was all about fun, and it was a lot of fun. I never said that I was going to become a veggie, or that I was going to get involved politically or become an activist; I was just going to have a good time and hang out with my movie star friend Woody Harrelson. But when I got out there on the road with those people, I started to see how their lifestyle affects who they are as individuals. I saw that when it comes to treating their bodies right, these people were serious, committed; they weren't just putting out some self-righteous bullshit line to make themselves feel superior to everybody else. And I saw how having that kind of commitment to your body really works; they had a glow in their eye, an alertness and an energy level that the vast majority of people just don't have.

You always hear the old saying, "You are what you eat," and those people I met on the SOL Tour really showed me how true that is. And when I started eating raw food with everybody else, I guess the same thing started happening to me without me even knowing it.

While my body was being transformed by the good food I was eating, being on the Tour was working on my brain as well. For my whole life to that point, I'd never taken an interest in politics or activist causes or any other shit like that, never even given it a moment's thought. I didn't really know anything about anything, except maybe music and weed. I'd always just lived in my own little world, having a blast with my friends, hanging by the seat of my pants, not caring about anything that

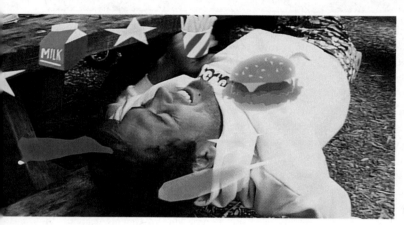

was going on outside of that little world. I would never stop to watch CNN or anything like that. I think the whole Gulf War thing started and ended before I even knew there was a problem over there. I think the country was already on its second George Bush before I realized there were two of them. I just didn't give a rat's ass.

But day after day on the SOL Tour, I listened to Woody and the others talk to students at the colleges along the way and to people we met along the road about the environment, deforestation, globalization, and corporate agriculture, and for the first time in my life it started to sink in. When I really started to listen, I just couldn't believe what I was hearing, and it pissed me off. As we drove past the acres and acres of clear-cut forest and the massive corporate farms, I started to see what was going on for the first time, and I found I was

getting more and more fired up about it every day. It also started to piss me off that so many people tend to dismiss activists like Woody and the other people on the SOL Tour as just pot-head yoga freaks, never stopping to actually listen to what they're saying. After a while, I started thinking, "Shit, these guys have a point about what's going on with the environment. We are losing control of our planet, and the evidence is all around us if we just open our eyes."

But I know there are lots of people out there who will never listen, not even for one minute. I saw that in the mixed feedback we got on the road. Most people were happy to see us and were interested in what Woody and his friends were talking about. But there were lots of people who called us freaks too, and some who even threw vegetables at our bus.

I'll admit, the Tour did manage to turn the light bulb on inside my head. And the sad truth is, it was a big stretch for a guy like me. I was always a person who lived for the moment, just gratifying my own immediate needs. In fact, I doubt you could ever find anybody who was more dedicated than me to doing just that. But as I became more aware of the problems, it really started to come home to me that, yeah, maybe I won't be on this planet forever, but there are lots of kids and future generations who will be here after I'm gone, and I need to show them some respect by the way I treat the planet. After all, it is the only one we've got and we've got to share it.

It's kind of like having a roommate who eats all your food and doesn't flush the toilet after he uses it and just kind of shrugs his shoulders and says, "Sorry man," but doesn't change his behavior. Well, I realized I was that kind of guy in the past but I didn't want to be that kind of guy anymore. That's one of the main things the SOL Tour did for me: it taught me to respect myself and to respect my fellow humans by respecting the planet. Plus, I learned that my individual actions do affect everybody else, which is something you don't even think about when you're caught up in your own little world.

I didn't know Woody that well before the SOL Tour. I mean, we hung out together on *Will & Grace* and partied together and stuff like that, but on the SOL Tour I really got to know the essence of what Woody is all about. He certainly talks the talk, and that puts a lot of people off right away because they don't always believe people like Woody actually live the way they encourage other people to live. Well, after spending a few weeks living on a bus with the man, I can honestly say he walks the walk better than anybody I know. He's really committed and passionate about his diet and his body and the planet, but not in a way that makes other people self-conscious about what they're doing. He's not afraid to speak out about his beliefs, but he's not a preacher. He just figures that if he does what he thinks is right and has the courage to speak about it, he might inspire other people to make changes in their lives that are going to benefit everybody.

I asked him a couple of times why he was doing it, why he would take time out to leave his home and go on the road, for no money, just to ask people to eat right and respect the planet. He just said he felt he had a duty to try, and if he managed to inspire just one person to make some changes, then it was worth it. Little did I know that I was one person of many in the course of that trip who would be inspired to walk, as they say, with "a lighter footprint on the earth."

The SOL Tour only lasted a few weeks, and it's been a few years since it happened, but I'm happy to say most of the changes I made in my life on that trip have been permanent. In fact, you could say I've officially joined the SOL tribe now. I mean, I'd call myself a vegetarian but I still can't quite do the raw food thing all the time. I also call myself an activist now and I'm aware of what's going on politically. I guess I'd have to say I'm engaged now, with myself and the planet, which is something I never was before. But that doesn't mean my entire personality has changed; I still look back at some of the people we ran into on the SOL Tour and think, "Man, what a granola-eating, sandal-wearing, incense-burning hippie fest that guy was."

I'm still nowhere near as hardcore as Woody when it comes to my diet, but I did pick up on some of his passion for healthy food. I don't go around preaching to anybody or anything like that, but I do try to let people know the things that I learned about eating right and healthy food. I guess I try to be an example to people that you don't necessarily have to be a hippie freak to eat organic and dig raw food. Lots of my old friends got in my face about the change in the beginning, but when they saw I was serious, they kind of sat back and listened a bit to what I was saying. And that's the best thing about it: being able to let people you care about

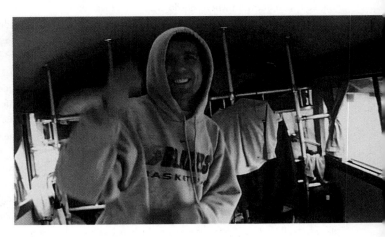

know some things that are going to help them live a better life. Like Woody, I figure if I can convince just one of my friends, by how healthy I am and through my passion for eating right, to give up the burgers and candy bars, then it's all worth it.

Actually, one of the most amazing things for me about the whole experience is the way the food I used to love makes me feel now. Now if I take even a bite of a Snickers bar or a Whopper my body almost goes into instant throw-up mode. It's like it has gotten so used to the good stuff that it says, "Shit Steve, what the hell is this you're givin' me?" It doesn't happen overnight, for sure. But over the course of weeks and months, when you gradually wean yourself off the meat, the dairy, and the sugar, you realize you're feeling better than you ever did in your life.

For me, the transformation was just amazing. I went from being this Deadhead guy working in Hollywood, smokin' weed, eatin' burgers, and listening to Peter Frampton, to opening my head a little bit and starting to use my brain. I was more alert and seeing things clearly for the first time, and I believe that was because I was eating living food. Suddenly I could see how I was supporting negative shit like corporate agriculture by eating food that wasn't any good for me anyway. Raw food is like some kind of natural benny actually—you feel so awake and so alive and you have so much energy. On top of that, you don't really get hungry that much because you're getting so much nutrition when you do eat. When I was eating crap, I'd get hungry and go to McD's or Wendy's or whatever and order the triple burger, which would hold me for maybe two or three hours and then I'd feel hungry again. That's because I wasn't really getting any nutrition; with the raw food you get nothing but nutrition.

I came out of the SOL Tour all inspired and fired up about my diet and the planet and everything else, and I'm still that way today. But I found out pretty fast that you can't just push that feeling on people if they're not open to it; you can't preach. I'll admit that I lost a few friends because of the changes that took place in me over the course of that trip down the coast. When I got back to Hollywood, the guys who were watching my dogs and my place had all kinds of frozen pizza and chicken and hamburgers in the fridge and I just freaked out when I saw it. I told them to get it the hell out of my house.

My friends just looked at me and said, "What the hell is up with you, man? A few weeks ago you were eatin' all this shit; half of it is yours anyway. Now you're gettin' in our face for doin' what you've been doin' your whole life, up until a few weeks ago."

They were right. I'll admit it: for a while after I came back from the SOL Tour I was out of control. In my worst moments, I even refused to talk to meat eaters. But I learned you can't judge people like that. They don't know; I didn't know either, until somebody filled me in. And I think that's what was so great about the SOL Tour: it showed people alternatives without making any judgments. That's what turns people off any time you try to show them a different way. That was probably the most important lesson I learned on the Tour: you can't tell people what to do because they have to make their own decisions about their own life. All you can do is be the best example you can be in the way you live. And I don't even consider myself an example; I'm just living my life in a way I now know is good for me and good for the planet.

Still, when my friends saw that I was serious about making some permanent changes in my life, I guess some of them didn't want to deal with it. I don't know if that's because they didn't like the new me or they didn't like the old them. It didn't matter though—I had to move on. Now I've got a whole new attitude about it all. Sometimes a friend will ask me in a restaurant if I mind if they order a steak and I tell them right away, "Hey man, you order what you want to order; don't worry about me. I don't want you to change your diet to suit me." But then I always add, "But, I'm telling you, when I changed my diet, I felt better than I ever did in my whole life." And I leave it at that.

But when people do ask me now about why I eat and think the way I do, I'm not afraid to let them know how I feel. And that's because we're never going to change the world for the better unless we voice ourselves whenever we get the chance. I just look at it like a chance to educate people about things that I was educated about by Woody and his friends, sort of passing on the knowledge, because people can't make informed choices if they're not informed. Like me, once they are informed about the alternatives, chances are they'll make the right choices. For instance, I don't know how people can continue to eat candy bars after they know the destruction all that refined sugar does to the body. And I don't know how they could continue to eat meat after they've seen what cows go through on their way to becoming a hamburger. That's really my prime motivation for not eating meat now. I love animals. I have had dogs all my life, and really, a cow isn't so different. I just decided I didn't want to eat anything that has a face anymore. I believe that cows have feelings and families and experience love, and we shouldn't be eating them with ketchup and mustard and a slice of cheese.

My attitude about the world has changed completely as well. Now I know what's going on in the world politically, socially, and economically, and I know who pulls the strings. I know what I need to do to stop being a part of the problem, and I can go to bed at night knowing that I've done my best to keep my money out of the hands of multinational corporations. I've done my best not to support corporate agriculture, unfair labor practices, and companies that harm the environment. In the end, that's all you can do.

It's true that I've lost friends because of my new diet and my new philosophy but it's also true that I've made a lot of new friends because of the changes I made. Now I know lots of people who are vegetarian, when before I don't think I knew a single one except Woody. And I've also met a lot of cool people who are environmental and political activists, so the world has opened up for me in a lot of different ways. It's like the SOL Tour is every day for me now.

I still slip a bit now and then on the candy and the chocolate, especially at Halloween and Christmas. But I think I can safely say that I'll never eat meat again. And I vote now, which is something I never did before because, like a lot of other people, I figured my vote wouldn't make a difference. Just think, if only a few thousand more people had thought their vote would make a difference, then maybe we could have avoided Bush II and all the problems that came with him. Now I know we have to vote, and if you don't, you're just making a conscious decision to let other people run the world they way they want. Now I believe you've got to voice yourself. If you don't, if you just let things go as they go, then your life is really kind of a waste.

If I had to pick my best memory from the SOL Tour, I'd have to say it's the feeling of love that surrounded that bus. That whole Tour was about love—love for each other and love for the earth. It was the time of my life, and I carry that feeling with me every day. We were like freedom fighters on a crusade for the planet, and it felt good. We felt the whole time like we were on a mission, and the mission was righteous. The whole message of the trip just felt right for everybody—eat right, treat the planet right, walk with a lighter footprint. It's simple but it works. And I know I'll spend the rest of my life being aware, living in the moment, and making a difference.

Go Further!

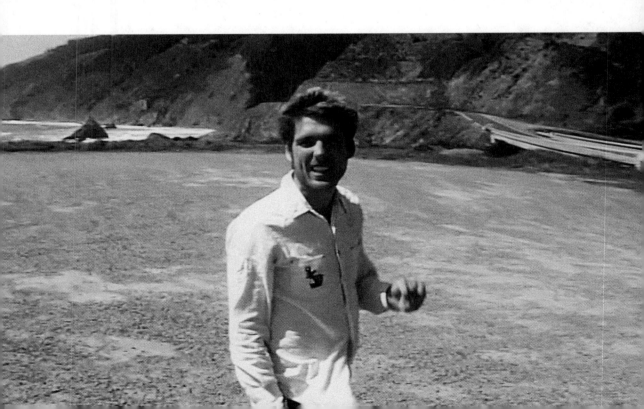

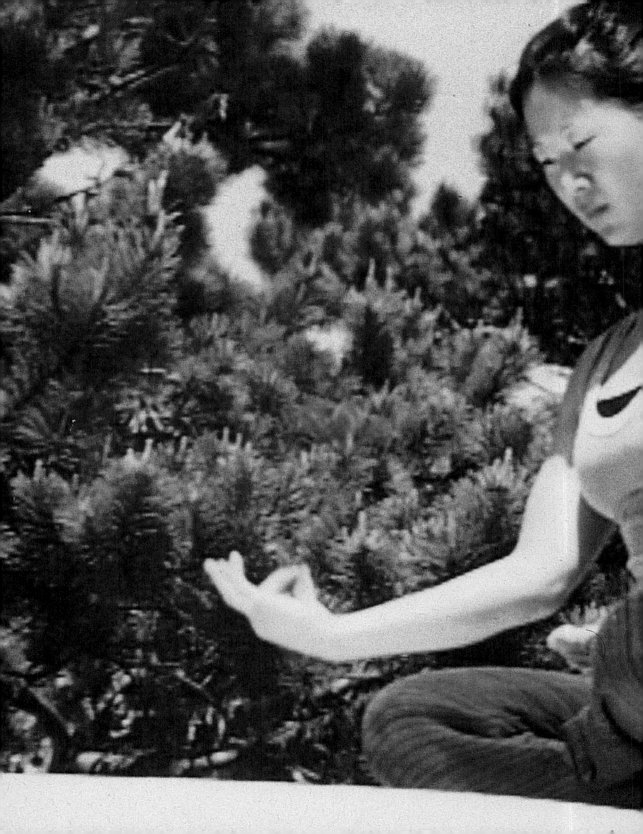

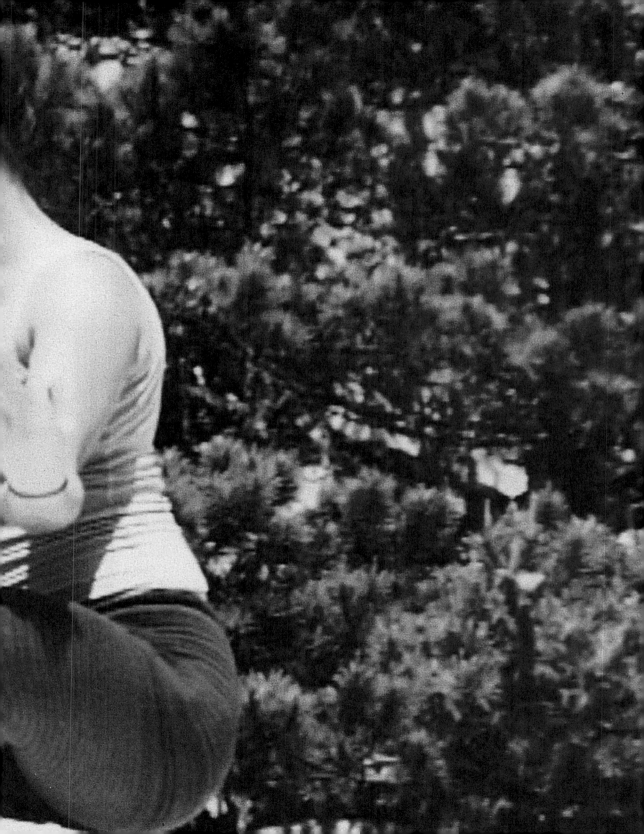

YOGA

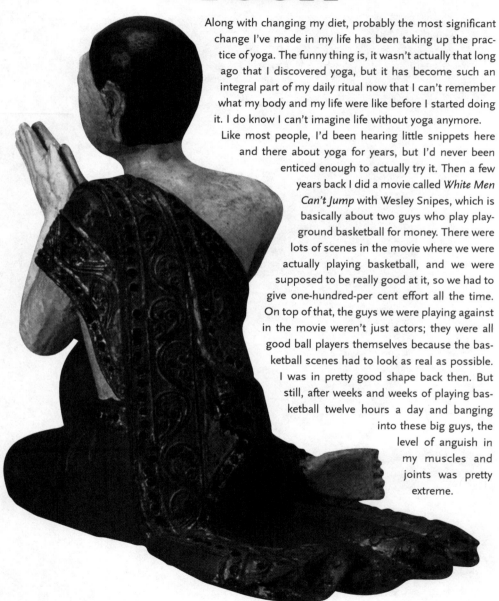

Along with changing my diet, probably the most significant change I've made in my life has been taking up the practice of yoga. The funny thing is, it wasn't actually that long ago that I discovered yoga, but it has become such an integral part of my daily ritual now that I can't remember what my body and my life were like before I started doing it. I do know I can't imagine life without yoga anymore.

Like most people, I'd been hearing little snippets here and there about yoga for years, but I'd never been enticed enough to actually try it. Then a few years back I did a movie called *White Men Can't Jump* with Wesley Snipes, which is basically about two guys who play playground basketball for money. There were lots of scenes in the movie where we were actually playing basketball, and we were supposed to be really good at it, so we had to give one-hundred-per cent effort all the time. On top of that, the guys we were playing against in the movie weren't just actors; they were all good ball players themselves because the basketball scenes had to look as real as possible. I was in pretty good shape back then. But still, after weeks and weeks of playing basketball twelve hours a day and banging into these big guys, the level of anguish in my muscles and joints was pretty extreme.

Wes and I were having so much fun playing with these guys on the set that we would still keep on playing even when the cameras weren't rolling, challenging one another and having little shooting and dribbling competitions between takes. On one particular night we were filming this scene where Wes and I had just won all this money in a basketball game and we get into an argument about whether or not I can slam-dunk the ball. My character gets really mad and then demands that they pull over at the next court and bets Wes's character his share of the money that he can dunk. Then he ends up losing it all.

Well, while Wes and I were shooting that scene, we actually did get into a real-life betting competition about me slamming the ball. The rims we used in the movie were set at nine-and-a-half feet, six inches lower than a regulation rim. But even so, I just couldn't get high enough to slam the ball. Each time I tried it, the bets would get higher and higher and I would get more and more frustrated when I couldn't do it.

Wes, of course, was having a great time with this. The whole crew was gathered around watching him dominate me in our little competition and he just lapped it up. Every time he would dunk it, everyone would cheer and he would strut around the court like he was God's gift to basketball. Then, when I failed, he would just laugh his ass off and go around high-fiving everybody. I finally gave up, and Wes swaggered off to his trailer having completely eviscerated the last vestiges of my athletic pride.

I sat on the court sulking, but the competition was far from over for me. First of all, I was pissed off that Wes had showed me up so badly in front of the whole crew. More than that though, as a life-long athlete and, I thought, a pretty good basketball player, I just couldn't accept that I couldn't slam the ball, especially with a lowered rim. Then this girl who was working on the crew as a boom operator came up to me and said, "If you want to jump higher, what you should do is stretch."

"What the hell," I thought; I had nothing else to do because it was going to take them about an hour to set up for the next scene, so I started stretching. At the beginning, I couldn't believe how tight my muscles had become, especially in my legs, after playing so much basketball. I stayed out there on the court for the next twenty minutes or so, just working every muscle and joint and getting everything loosened up again. Finally, when I felt ready, I put some sticky stuff on my hand, picked up the ball, took a good long run at the rim, and slammed it.

What is Yoga?

THE PRACTICE OF YOGA CAN BE DEFINED IN TWO VERY DISTINCT WAYS. IN THE EAST, YOGA IS AN ANCIENT HINDU DISCIPLINE DESIGNED TO MOVE THE INDIVIDUAL TOWARD A STATE OF TRANQUILITY, PEACE OF MIND, AND SPIRITUAL ENLIGHTENMENT. TO THOSE WHO FOLLOW YOGA RELIGIOUSLY, SUCH AS DEVOUT HINDUS AND BUDDHISTS, THE GOAL OF THE PRACTICE IS TOTAL UNION WITH BRAHMAN (OR THE ABSOLUTE) AND ATMAN (THE TRUE SELF). IN WESTERN CULTURES, HOWEVER, YOGA IS USUALLY THOUGHT OF AS SIMPLY A SYSTEM OF PHYSICAL EXERCISES THAT PEOPLE USE TO GAIN CONTROL OF THEIR BODY AND IMPROVE THEIR OVERALL FITNESS.

THE WORD "YOGA" COMES FROM THE SANSKRIT WORD "YUJ," WHICH MEANS UNION. (ALONG WITH PALI, SANSKRIT IS ONE OF THE LANGUAGES OF ANCIENT INDIA AND IS THE LANGUAGE OF MANY HINDU AND BUDDHIST HOLY TEXTS.) THE PRACTICE OF YOGA CAN BE TRACED BACK TO THE INDUS-SARAVATI CIVILIZATION THAT FLOURISHED IN INDIA ABOUT 5000 YEARS AGO. THE PRINCIPLES OF YOGA WERE FIRST WRITTEN DOWN BY A HINDU TEACHER NAMED PATANJALI, WHO BROUGHT THEM TOGETHER IN A RELIGIOUS SCRIPTURE KNOWN AS THE *YOGA SUTRA*. OVER THE CENTURIES, SEVERAL NEW FORMS OF YOGA WERE CREATED, EACH FOCUSING ON A DIFFERENT ASPECT OF PERSONAL DEVELOPMENT. DURING THE 1920s, HATHA YOGA WAS POPULARIZED THROUGHOUT THE WEST BY A TEACHER NAMED T. KRISHNAMACHAKYATHE, AND IT REMAINS THE MOST POPULAR FORM OF YOGA TODAY.

EVEN THOUGH IT IS CLOSELY ASSOCIATED WITH THE EASTERN RELIGIONS, YOGA ITSELF IS NOT A RELIGION. THERE ARE MANY PEOPLE WHO STILL PRACTICE YOGA FOR RELIGIOUS REASONS TODAY, PRIMARILY IN INDIA, BUT THE MAJORITY OF MODERN PRACTITIONERS DO IT SIMPLY TO STAY FIT. ONE OF THE MAIN REASONS WHY YOGA HAS BECOME SUCH A POPULAR FITNESS OPTION IS BECAUSE THERE ARE VIRTUALLY NO PHYSICAL BARRIERS TO PARTICIPATION; THE HEIGHT, WEIGHT, SEX, AGE, AND GENDER OF THE PRACTITIONER IS IRRELEVANT, AND THE ONLY EQUIPMENT REQUIRED IS LOOSE CLOTHING AND AN EXERCISE MAT.

UNLIKE OTHER FORMAL PHYSICAL EXERCISE, YOGA IS PROCESS-ORIENTED. THE IDEA IS NOT TO FOCUS ON WHAT YOU *WANT TO DO*, BUT ON *WHAT YOU ARE DOING* AND *HOW YOU FEEL WHILE DOING IT*. PHYSICAL TRAINING TENDS TO BREAK DOWN AND REBUILD MUSCLES, WHEREAS YOGA TONES THEM INSTEAD. IN ADDITION, RESEARCH SHOWS THAT THE STRETCHING AND BREATHING EXERCISES OF YOGA CAN HELP WITH ASTHMA, EPILEPSY, ANXIETY AND STRESS. THEY ALSO HELP MAKE THE PRACTITIONER MORE RELAXED, INCREASE CONCENTRATION, AND TAKE TOXINS OUT OF THE BODY. YOGA MAY EVEN HELP PEOPLE LIVE LONGER.

—KH.

After I did it, I just stood there stunned for a couple of seconds. Then, just to make sure I hadn't dreamed it all, I picked up the ball and slammed it again. It was clear right then that just twenty minutes of stretching had loosened up my muscles enough that they were able to push me that much higher into the air; it was like the benefits of having the loose, flexible body that yoga creates were immediately evident. I was just amazed by that, and I was also psyched because now I knew I could slam the ball.

So I just kept stretching and smiling to myself as I waited for Wes to come out of his trailer. When he finally did come out, still all smug from his victory, I went right up to him and challenged him to double-or-nothing on our last bet. He tried to laugh me off and said he didn't want to take any more of my money, but eventually I wore him down and he finally said, "OK, man. If you want to lose again that bad . . ."

So the word went out and a crowd began to gather around the court again. Wes kept jawing at me about how crazy I was as I re-tied my shoelaces, and then I casually went over and picked up the ball. I waited at mid-court for a few seconds to let the tension build, then took off for the basket. I just flew down the court, and as I lifted off my feet just past the free-throw line, I could actually feel the difference in my body; before I stretched, my body felt like it was heavier and slower, but now I felt like I was moving twice as fast as before and that I could jump to the top of the backboard if I had to. This time I jumped higher than I had all day and slammed the ball with ease. The crew cheered wildly and Wes howled in amazement; he could not believe what he had just seen. He never did pay off the bet, but the look on his face was more than worth it.

After that experience, I became a lot more curious about the benefits of stretching and flexibility and that curiosity led me to the practice of yoga. Through friends I eventually got hooked up with this great yogi named Nateshfar and started to study yoga seriously. Once I got into it, I began to feel a kind of peacefulness that I had never experienced before. Almost immediately, yoga dispelled any anxiety I was feeling about my life and totally reset my clock.

It took some getting used to, of course, because it was so alien from the sports and fitness training I had grown up with. In Western society, we tend to come at physical activities from the "yang" perspective, the male side, where it's more about strength. Yoga, obviously, comes from the Eastern perspective and is much more "yin," the feminine side, focusing more on concentration and flexibility. But I soon found out it takes just as much strength—maybe more—to perform yoga as it does to perform any of the physical activities I'd been doing all my life.

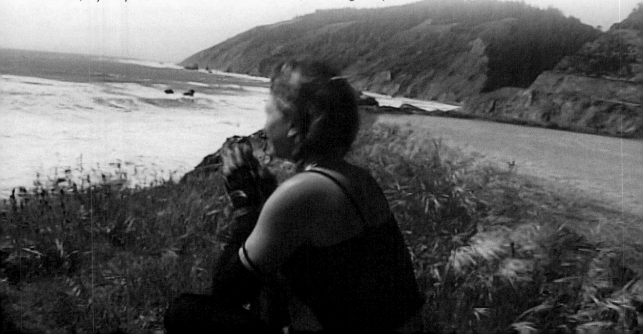

I guess it was right around then that I got hooked. I thought to myself: "Man, I thought I was fit, but this shit takes more strength and endurance than anything I've done before." And not only that, it was obvious that yoga also built up a kind of mental discipline that I found really fascinating. I sat looking at the instructor, sitting there smiling on his mat with his foot behind his head, gently encouraging the class without a hint of stress in his voice, and I thought, "I've gotta have that. What ever it is he's got, I've gotta have that." So right then I offered my body up on the altar of yoga, and I've been "born again" physically and mentally ever since.

It wasn't like I didn't know anything at all about yoga before I had my first class. Like most people, I knew it as some kind of exercise regimen from the East that involved tying your body in knots, and I knew the hippies really got into it in the 1960s. Well, I did some reading after my first class and I learned that the practice of yoga started in India about 5,000 years ago among mystics who were looking for a way to achieve better health and heightened self-awareness through physical and mental exercise. The whole idea was to bring the body and mind together in a perfectly harmonious state of being. In fact, the word "yoga" actually means "to join together."

It was a surprise for me to learn that there are more than a hundred schools or styles of yoga. They are all a little different and no one kind is better than any other; each one just has its own special focus depending on its founder or the instructor. Some of the most common styles are Ananda, which is the gentle, stretching yoga you see ladies doing in the church basement; Ashtanga, which is a more demanding, aerobic style that involves moving quickly through a series of difficult positions; and Bikram, which is like Ashtanga performed in a sauna—the goal of Bikram is to rid the body of toxins by sweating them out. Regardless of the specific focus of a particular yoga style, they all incorporate three central elements: exercise, breathing control, and meditation.

The exercise aspect of yoga, or the asana, comprises a series of positions you have to put your body in and hold, called postures. Each posture is designed to put pressure on your muscles, joints and tendons to build up flexibility, stamina, and strength. Lots of the postures are really uncomfortable at first but that's the whole idea. As a beginner you're expected to fight to maintain the posture; that gets you concentrating on your body, thinking about each muscle, joint, and tendon, working to keep control over them all.

The next key element of yoga is called pranayama, a releasing of the tensions of the mind. The focus is on breathing control. Oxygen is the very source of life in the body, and pranayama is designed to help you take control of your breathing so that you're always getting all the oxygen you need and using it with maximum efficiency. That made perfect sense to me as a sports lover—your body and mind can't function at their optimum level unless you're taking in enough oxygen, and that's especially true when your body is under stress. So the postures and the breathing control are linked, requiring you to maintain a certain breathing level or number of breaths for each posture.

It gets easier with practice, and eventually you'll start to feel it all coming together. You'll feel the tension leaving your body and you'll stop fighting the postures. Just like magic, things that were hard to do will seem effortless.

Of course, like all good things, it doesn't happen overnight. For starters, it takes your body a little while just to figure out what the hell is going on. Lots of people spend years using their body to do just a limited set of things—they sit in the same seat in the car; they stand or sit in the same place at work and perform the same tasks over and over, whether that's typing or writing or hammering nails. But yoga makes you do things with your body you've never asked it to do before. When you start to do yoga consistently, your brain suddenly starts to get new messages from your body: "We need to extend this tendon over here

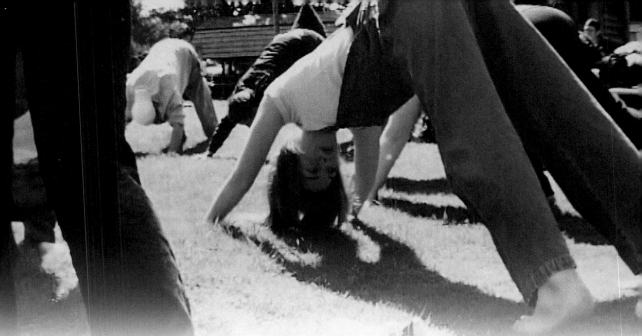

in the shoulder," "We need more muscle down here in the quads," "We need to burn some fat off this butt."

If the messages keep coming, the brain eventually responds, sending the right cells to the right place to remove all the crap the body doesn't need. Your muscles literally start to grow longer; your tendons become more flexible; your joints start to move more freely. All it takes is just a little bit every day. You can start with fifteen minutes, then bump that up to half an hour, then an hour. When you start, maybe you won't be able to touch your toes, but believe me, if you keep moving just a little bit farther every day, eventually you'll have your foot behind your head.

Once you gain mastery over your body, you'll find that you can do some amazing things you never would've thought you could do. And if you've got control of your breathing too, then you can remain just as cool, calm and collected in a difficult posture as you would be at home in your favorite armchair. The first goal of yoga is to gain that control, and once you've got it, you are set for the following stages, the stages of the mind: concentration, meditation, and, in the end, spiritual consciousness. That's what the ancient mystics were shooting for anyway. I haven't got there yet, but I figure I'm well on my way.

Probably the best thing about yoga for me is the fact that it's something I can take with me on my journey through life, however long that might be. That's important, because I don't know that good health is necessarily a pinnacle that anyone can reach; I see good health as more of a process that never ends, like the ongoing maintenance process that keeps your car on the road year after year. Your body is the vehicle that has to transport you through your life, and you're not going to get very far if your vehicle's got two flat tires and no gas.

You have to keep in mind that every day each one of us is bombarded by toxins and other negative influences in our environment. There's smog in the air and chemicals in the water and food; stress at work and at home; death and destruction on TV every night. Let's face it, all of that shit has got to take a toll on the body and mind eventually.

As well as all that, there are emotional issues that inevitably come up that are hard to deal with. Often, we don't deal with them at all. Maybe you get mad at somebody you care about, or a relationship breaks up, or you lose a job, or you get a speeding ticket. Lots of us tend to ball that negative energy up and push it way down inside ourselves where it blocks up our spirit and saps our positive energy. Every little thing that happens makes us hunch our shoulders a bit more, makes our stomach tighten a bit more.

The Eight Yogic Limbs

Every form of yoga is said to have eight limbs. These limbs are like stepping stones, and practitioners must concentrate on mastering one limb at a time as they work toward the goal of mastering all eight.

1. YAMA—Yama focuses on mastering ethical principles such as non-violence, truth, sharing, and self-control. People who practice yoga must try to apply these principles to every aspect of their lives.

2. NIYAMA—Niyama also involves self-discipline and focuses on the spiritual side of the yoga practitioner. It encourages the individual to take the time to worship a higher power and to practice meditation on a regular basis.

3. ASANA—Asana involves actual physical activity and is the best known aspect of the yoga lifestyle. The yogic disciple must practice postures regularly in order to master Asana.

4. PRANAYAMA—Pranayama uses techniques to train the mind to control breathing. Yoga sees a connection between the mind and how the body breathes, therefore this limb is designed to teach practitioners to take control of their breathing in order to better focus their mind.

5. PRATYAHARA—Here, practitioners are encouraged to go to a quiet place where they can meditate or perform postures. This place can be physical, or it can be a place created in the mind. In this place, they can better concentrate and reflect upon their life, free of outside distractions.

6. DHARANA—Dharana is the sixth limb, and it focuses on meditation itself. Dharana trains the mind to rid itself of distractions during meditation, such as unnecessary noises, thoughts and ideas. Mastering Dharana is very difficult and requires a great deal of patience and discipline from the yoga practitioner. Most individuals living in our modern society are use to being bombarded constantly with sensory stimuli, and therefore find it almost impossible, at first, to "switch off" their senses and clear their mind completely. This is the goal of Dharana.

7. DHYANA—Dhyana is the seventh limb. By the time they reach this stage, the yoga practitioner will be able to meditate with absolutely no distractions. When a person has achieved dhyana, their mind is quiet, their body in total control, and they develop the ability to be aware of what they are doing without concentrating. Dhyana can best be described as "living effortlessly", and only the most devoted practitioners reach this stage.

8. SAMADHI—The very last yogic limb is somewhat similar to the Buddhist concept of enlightenment or nirvana. When a yoga practitioner reaches Samadhi, they are said to have completely connected with god, and their self no longer matters.

–KH.

I don't think you need to be a genius to figure out that this is no way to live, although so many people choose to. The fact is, if you don't find some way of releasing all the negative energy in your life, and some way of expelling all the toxins in your body, eventually they'll eat you up. And that's just what yoga is designed to do: to release that negative energy, to restore vitality and peace to your body, mind, and soul. In that way, yoga can be a life-long healer.

So whenever anybody asks me why I'm so committed to yoga, I always tell them that, for me, it's really a quality-of-life issue. It's certainly not about *quantity* of life; I don't need to live to be 200 years old, but I would like to spend the time that I have left in a vehicle that can take me where I want to go. I know I can never regain my lost youth, but I still want to keep my body healthy enough to house my youthful spirit.

I believe achieving that goal is more than possible for all of us, and I believe yoga can help anybody get there. What yoga does, ultimately, is make the impossible possible. It makes you see that, with a little effort, you can do things with your body and mind that you never knew you could do. And once you realize you can have that kind of control over your body and mind, you can carry that feeling over into other parts of your life. That's how you achieve inner peace.

So that's why I encourage everyone I meet to try yoga—because I want people to realize themselves more fully, the way I feel I have. I want people to feel something more than they are used to feeling, because I know there's so much more than that.

You know, those ancient Indian mystics were on to something. I've found it really is true that when you become genuinely aware of what's going on inside you, you can begin to become more engaged in the world around you and, eventually, more connected to the world beyond this one.

It's really simple when you think about it: connect with yourself, connect with your environment, connect with God.

Yoga—to join together. Body. Mind. Spirit.

So now that you know where you're going, pull up a mat and let's get started . . .

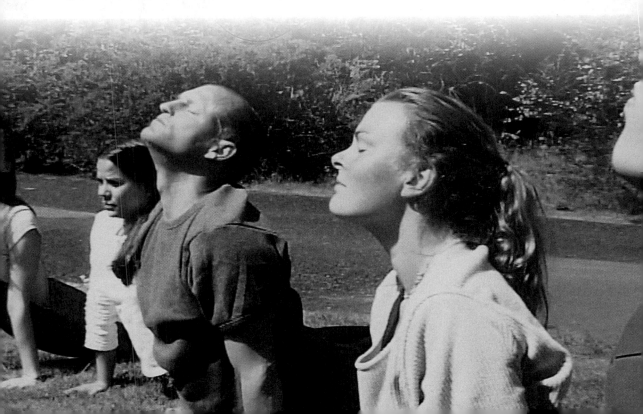

RESEARCH

NO TRES

PROPERTY

PASSING

AGRICULTURE

Whenever I talk to people about the things I believe in, someone always asks me what I think is the most significant thing you can do to help improve the health of the planet. Well, without question, I believe the most important thing we can do to help the planet, and to help ourselves for that matter, is to take a look at our diet. And, ultimately, that means making the switch to organic.

If you go back just seventy years, to before World War II, basically all the food consumed in the world was produced by family farmers using age-old farming methods that today we would call "organic." After the war though, Western societies got sucked in by the notion that science and technology could improve crop yields, and we started to ignore all that was good about the way we used to do things.

By the 1970s, we were pumping more than 450,000 tons of pesticides on our crops every year in the United States alone. The crap we spray on our fruits and vegetables actually acts in much the same way radiation does to kill bugs and fungus, except it would take something like 145 H-bombs to achieve the same deadly effect worldwide. Yet most people don't even question the use of chemicals on fruits and vegetables.

Today the family farm is almost a thing of the past. In the 1900 U.S. census, about fifty per cent of the population were dependent on farming for at least some, if not all, of their personal income. Now, just over a century later, only about one per cent of the population of the United States considers themselves farmers. Pretty soon it won't even be worth having a box on the census form for farmer. The Old MacDonald we all like to think of, with his traditional way of life and his deep connection to the land, has been overrun by corporate agribusiness, with its factory farms, pesticides, herbicides, hormones, and

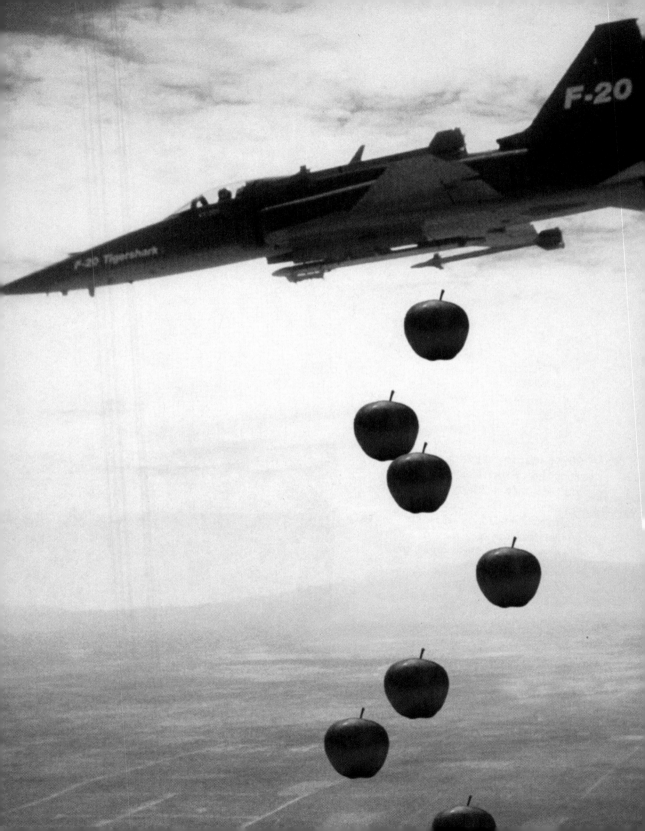

In 1999, the Consumers Union used data from the USDA's Pesticide Data Program to compare the relative amounts and toxicity of pesticide residues in various foods to determine a "relative toxicity loading" of each. The foods with the highest toxicity loading were

- fresh peaches (both U.S.-grown and imported)
- frozen and fresh winter squash (U.S.-grown)
- apples (U.S.-grown and imported)
- grapes (U.S.-grown and imported)
- spinach (U.S.-grown and imported)
- pears (U.S.-grown and imported)
- green beans (U.S.-grown)

Source: Edward Groth et al. Do You Know What You're Eating?

genetic modification. The corporate farming people argue that all this scientific and technological progress has improved food production and quality. I'm not so sure—not when one in every three people gets cancer and one out of every two develops heart disease.

Now that only one per cent of the population of the United States is involved in farming, it has to make you wonder how that paradigm shift has altered the perspective of the generations of people who grew up in the cities and the sprawling suburbs. Our modern society has become so separated from the land that I wonder how many people really understand anymore the basic ecological functions of water and soil, of animals, plants, and insects. In fact, most of us today have no connection to the land at all.

If each one of us just stopped to think about it for a minute, most people would realize we don't really know where our food comes from, how it is produced, and by whom. And if we took the time to look into it, we probably wouldn't like what we found. In fact, I'm sure if the average person were to take a tour of a corporate hog farm, he or she would never eat another piece of bacon again.

I've noticed that when people learn the truth about how most of our food is produced today, their expression changes; they instinctively know that the current situation is just not right. In their hearts, I think people realize that factory farming is not going to be the answer in the long term because it's just not sustainable. We are exhausting the soil by pumping it full of chemicals it can't absorb and trying to raise thousands of animals on farms where they used to raise a few hundred.

There's a serious crisis brewing in the world and the cause is widespread ecological ignorance. The forces of corporate agribusiness are poised to take over our food supply, and they've been able to do it because people have lost touch with the planet. The only way to stop this is for each one of us to become an active participant in determining our diet—deciding not only what we eat but also how it's produced and who produces it. I believe if you really want to help the planet, you have to start by reconnecting with the land, and the best way to do that is to go organic.

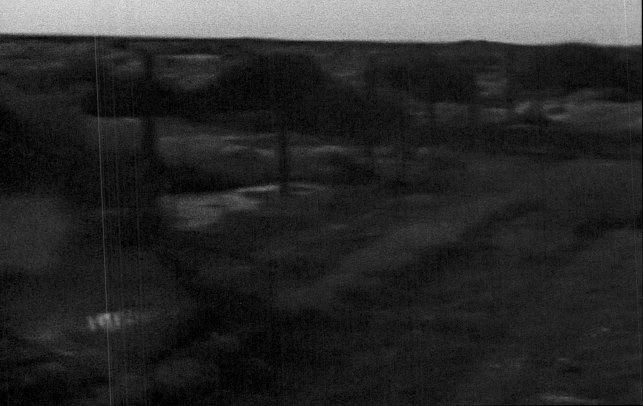

Chemical Farming

Our journey down the West Coast took us past the massive factory farms of Northern California, and I had to cover my mouth and nose more than a few times as the crop dusters flew overhead, spraying their poison on anything and everything for miles downwind. In fact, I'm reminded of that experience every time I go to the market to buy organically grown fruit and vegetables, because organic farmers have to make a special effort to make sure people know that they don't do that to their produce.

Anyone who buys organically grown fruits and vegetables knows they usually come covered with stickers—from the farmer, from the growers' co-operative, from the organic certification organizations. The stickers are there to assure customers that the apples or cobs of corn haven't been sprayed, nuked, or genetically altered on the way to their table. On the other hand, "conventional" fruit and vegetables grown on factory farms usually don't come with any stickers at all, unless it's the company logo. It seems the agri-corporations can promote their produce as "healthy" and "natural," but they don't have

to slap a warning on there that says "irradiated," "genetically modified," or "treated with chemicals."

That just demonstrates to me how screwed up our priorities have become when it comes to the food we eat. We live in a world today where customers need to be told when a piece of fruit or a vegetable was grown without chemical or genetic interference. But take something that was grown from a seed created in a laboratory, coat it with all kinds of shit from someone's chemistry set, and that is what we now call conventional produce. The word "conventional" means standard, ordinary, typical. But today, if you take a normal apple seed, plant it in the ground, and grow a tree using nothing but clear water and sunlight, then pick the apples and take them to market, those apples are no longer standard, ordinary, or typical. Suddenly they're something different: they're "organic" apples, and they need to have a sticker or two, so you can tell them apart from the Frankenfruit. It's a topsy-turvy world, there's no doubt about it.

Actually, pesticides and herbicides have been around long enough now that we really should know better. It all started back before World War I when scientists figured out how to synthetically alter the levels of nutrients that

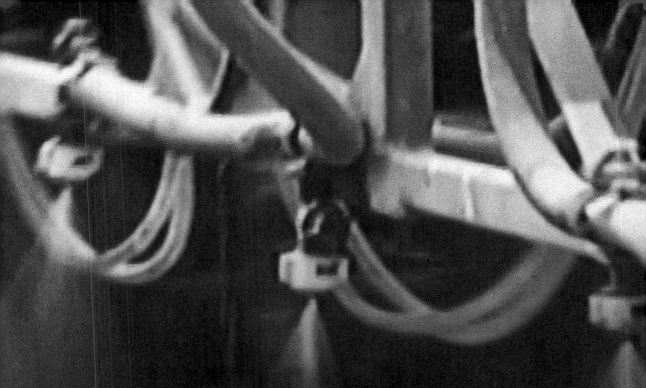

are naturally in the soil, such as potassium, phosphorus, and nitrogen, to get bigger plants and better yields. But when some yields started to get so big the farmers couldn't maintain the plants, the scientists had to find ways to kill bugs and weeds on a larger scale. They found that modern chemicals were good for that too, but they didn't stop to think about what would happen when the chemicals seeped into the groundwater where they could be ingested by livestock and, eventually, live people too.

By the time they realized that the shit they were spraying on the plants could have an enormous effect on people, animals, and whole ecosystems, it was too late. Manufacturing pesticides and herbicides had become a big business, and most of the farmers got hooked on the stuff because they thought they could make more money using it. I don't blame the farmers though; all they ever wanted to do was make a living. Meanwhile, the chemical companies were feeding them the same line about pesticides and herbicides that they were feeding the public: they're perfectly safe; they'll improve your yield; you'll get a better price for your crop. When the factory farms started pushing the family farmers into bankruptcy, using chemicals became a matter of survival.

Of course, our elected representatives could have stepped in when they realized that pouring chemicals into the food supply wasn't a good idea, but politicians are usually not in a hurry to piss off either the farmers or the chemical companies. So the politicians basically crossed their fingers and hoped for the best. In truth, we all put our faith in science and technology and corporate leaders. There was a time, from after World War II right up through the 60s, when we really believed that science and technology were going to lead us to the Promised Land. By now we were all supposed to be going around in flying cars and modern chemicals were going to make food so abundant and nutritious that no one would ever go hungry. "Peace through science," they said.

It didn't exactly work out like that though, did it? In fact, a lot of things the government and the corporations have told us over the years didn't work out at all like they said they would. Remember the pesticide DDT that was sprayed all over playgrounds and public parks to kill mosquitoes? The chemical companies used to say you could drink it. And what about Agent Orange? They told the soldiers in Vietnam that it would only kill plants. We know better now. But do we?

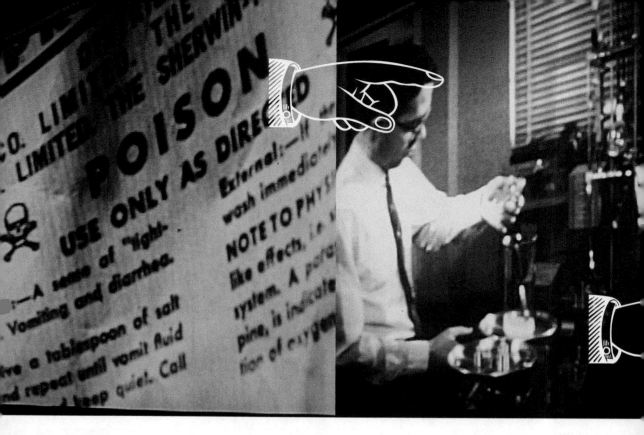

Genetically Engineered Food

I believe we are going down exactly the same path today with genetically engineered (GE) food that we went down with pesticides and herbicides sixty years ago. Just as the chemical companies did then, the agri-corporations are telling us we have nothing to fear from GE food; they've done the research, they say, and they've got it all under control. Well, if we've been paying attention, history should tell us to start worrying any time big business says they've got everything under control. They may be able to prove that GE food won't kill anybody who eats it today, but they can't say for sure that GE food won't have a negative effect on people ten, twenty, or thirty years from now.

How can any scientist say for sure what happens when you introduce a transgenic crop (meaning a crop that has genetic material from another species—in other words, an alien life form) into a finely balanced ecosystem? They may know that if they add a particular genome to a certain plant, it will be able to better protect itself from insects, for example. But what happens when those insects start to disappear? What effect will taking away the insects have on birds and animals that need those insects to survive? And on the animals that eat those animals? Altering the genetic makeup of a cash crop may solve one problem for agribusiness but it will have other consequences down the food chain that won't show up for years, or even decades.

While genetic modification may be pretty new stuff, it's not like we don't have enough past examples of what happens when you mess with nature to make us think twice about it. English settlers introduced rabbits to Australia in the nineteenth century because they liked to hunt them. But without enough natural predators to control their population, the rabbits did what rabbits do best, and now the Australian continent has got a huge rabbit infestation problem. The zebra mussel is another example; it was transported to the Great Lakes from the other side of the world in wastewater brought by cargo

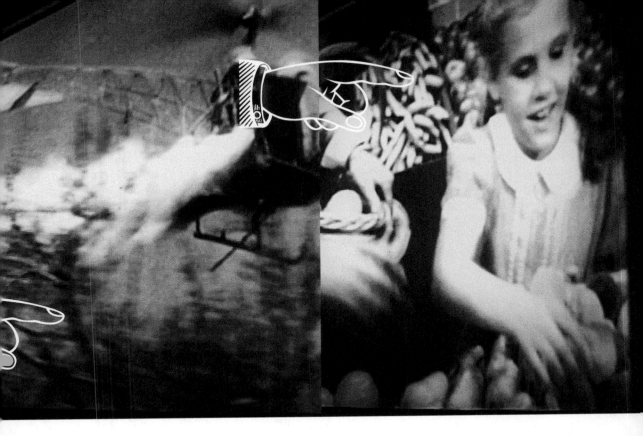

ships decades ago. Now scientists say the Great Lakes are dying because there are so many zebra mussels that there isn't enough oxygen in the water for the fish. The scientists call it "invasion biology." Of ten foreign species that are introduced into a new ecosystem, maybe only one will survive, but the one species that does manage to survive could have a devastating effect on that ecosystem, changing it forever. We roll that dice with each new bio-engineered species we introduce into our ecosystem. So can the agri-corporations really say that there is nothing to worry about with GE food? If they want to be honest about it, I think it's pretty obvious that they can't.

Anyway, why the hell should we believe these corporations when they are fighting like hell to make sure consumers don't even have the right to know whether or not products use genetically engineered ingredients? When you buy a can of frozen juice, the company that made it can print "all-natural flavors" on the label (whatever that means) but there's no law that forces them to

print "Made with genetically altered, non-organic fruit."

In 2000, a coalition of activist groups, including the Pesticide Action Network and Friends of the Earth, pooled their resources and had some tests done on some taco shells that were sold through grocery stores under the Taco Bell brand name. They found that the taco shells contained a transgenic corn with the trademarked name StarLink that is not approved for human consumption by the U.S. Food and Drug Administration (FDA); it's supposed to be used strictly for non-food industrial purposes and as feed corn for livestock. When the groups came forward with their research, the owner of the StarLink patent, the multinational pharmaceutical company Aventis, challenged the findings. Since the corporations weren't going to do anything about it, the FDA was basically forced to step in and do its own tests, and it ended up finding that there was, in fact, StarLink corn in the taco shells.

If that comes as a shock to you, it shouldn't; crap like that is standard operating procedure in corporate

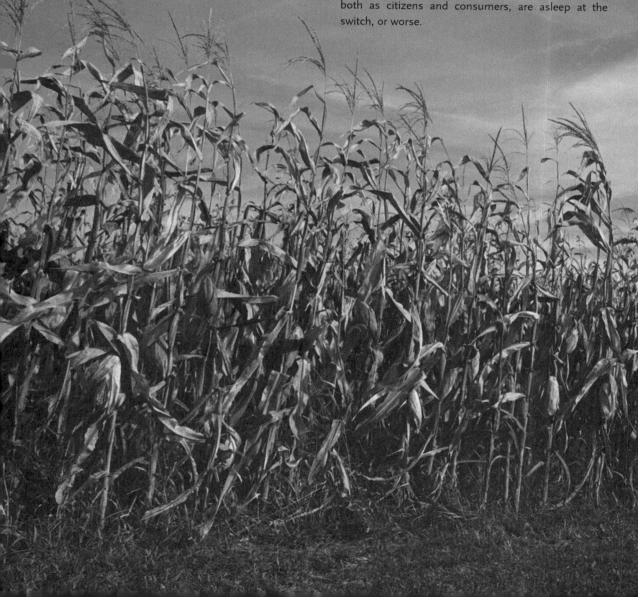

America. But I do think things like the StarLink controversy should be enough to wake people up to the fact that we need to become more aware of what's going on with our food supply. The scary thing about it is that if those concerned citizens' groups hadn't looked into it on their own, people still wouldn't know they were eating, and paying top price for, cheap GE feed corn.

I think it's high time we woke up to the fact we are living in a world where huge corporations are doing nasty things to the food we eat and other huge corporations are selling us that food at the grocery store and the drive-thru. Often these are the same corporations that brought us DDT and Agent Orange, and now they're breaking into the very genetic fabric of life. Who made them God, is what I'd like to know. And if you don't believe they're playing God, then at the very least they're conducting a giant unchecked scientific experiment with our planet. Meanwhile, the politicians and regulatory agencies that are supposed to protect us, both as citizens and consumers, are asleep at the switch, or worse.

Hidden Agenda

If you're not particularly concerned about what tampering with the genetic codes of the foods we eat could mean for your health, you should be concerned about what it could mean for the future of our society. Throughout history, power has always been directly related to the control of essential resources: water, energy, raw materials and, most importantly, food. The societies that were the most successful at developing and harnessing these resources flourished, while the ones that couldn't provide for their people were either conquered or simply disappeared. I believe that the multinational agri-corporations want to take control of the global food supply, and genetic engineering is how they plan to do it.

The idea that a person or a company can own a living thing is obviously not a new one: you own your pets and the trees in your yard; farmers own their livestock and the crops in their fields. But the idea that a person or a company can own a certain *type* of living thing, be it a certain variety of a vegetable, or a certain breed of animal, outright and not just for now but forever, is terrifying. Sadly, that is exactly where the insanity of genetic engineering is leading us.

There's nothing simple about the science behind genetic engineering, but it's not too hard to see how the agri-corps plan to use it to hold our food supply for ransom. Take corn for example. Corn is one of the most important food crops and the fourth most widely grown crop in the world. The corn varieties we know today are actually descended from wild grasses that had tiny, barely edible kernels. It took thousands of years of Native Indian subsistence farmers replanting seeds from plants with the biggest, sweetest, juiciest kernels in order for corn to evolve into the plant we know today. There are lots of varieties of corn, all developed naturally, and none of them belongs to anybody; they are a gift from our ancestors and belong to all of us. But Monsanto, a huge agri-corp based in St. Louis, Missouri, doesn't see it that way.

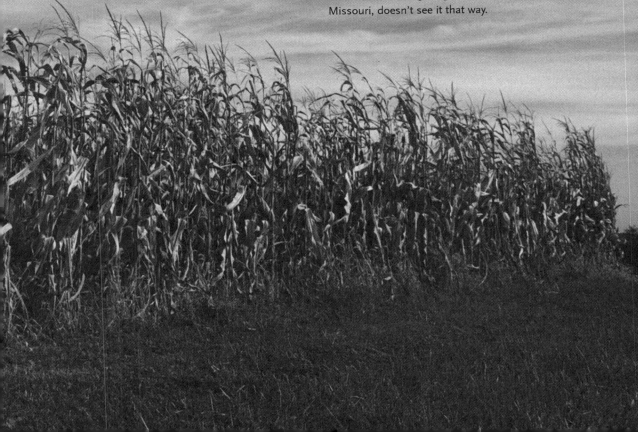

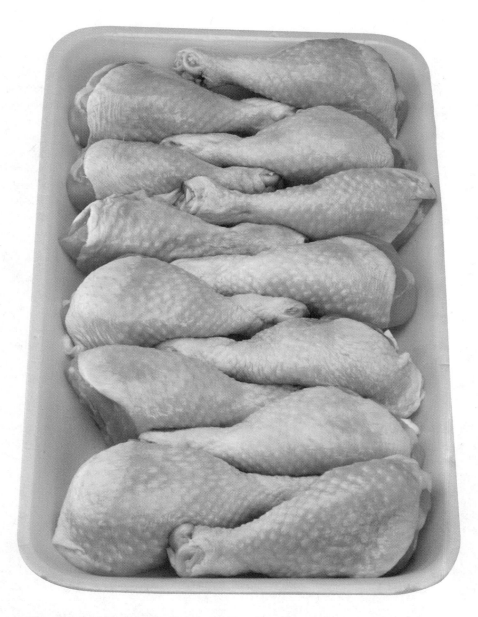

Five corporations—IBP, Conagra, Cargill, Farmland National Beef, Packerland Packing Co.—control 79 per cent of the American beef packing industry, and four companies control over 50 per cent of the poultry processing industry. Through mergers and acquisitions, these companies have managed to vertically integrate the entire process, owning not only the farms where the animals are raised, but also the slaughterhouses and packing plants as well.

Source: Tad Williams, <u>The Corruption of American Agriculture.</u>

On the pretext of controlling a little bug called the corn borer, Monsanto took a naturally occurring, or heirloom, variety of corn and modified its genetic code in the laboratory so that it would produce high levels of a natural pesticide called *Bacillus thuringiensis*. The result, called Bt corn, pumps this toxin out of every cell, from the root to the stalk to the corn kernels themselves. Well, not only can Bt corn kill the corn borer, it kills any insect that tries to feed on it, keeping the cobs nice and pretty for the grocery store. Monsanto says it's a wonderful thing for farmers and consumers because it cuts down on the amount of pesticide that has to be used to control the pests. That's true. But it cuts down on other pests too, like corn farmers who choose not to plant it.

The problem with genetically engineered crops like Bt corn is that they don't care who they have sex with. When the corn waves in the wind, its pollen is taken up and travels for miles in all directions, free to cross-pollinate any plant it lands on. If some of the pollen from the Bt corn pollinates organically grown corn on another farm, its specific genetic signature will show up in the DNA of the next generation of organic corn, and that creates a couple of problems. First of all, the cross-pollinated organic corn is now genetically modified as well. Second, Monsanto happens to own the patent on the genetic signature for Bt corn containing Monsanto event 80, and since the organic farmer didn't pay the license fee to Monsanto for the privilege of planting their Bt corn seed, he is effectively stealing their product.

It's a pretty neat trick. What Monsanto and the other corporate agriculture giants have done through the genetic engineering of food crops is take something that was a common asset and turn it into their intellectual property. They say they're creating these genetic mutations for the most altruistic reasons, but it's all driven by profit. They say they are introducing more varieties, but their goal is actually the opposite: to achieve homogeneity. If they own the rights to the genetic code of a crop that is free to spread that code to other similar varieties, eventually the other varieties will be wiped out. You can't control the spread of plant DNA like it's an oil spill. And once the new genetic code is implanted, you can't just take it out. So if a family farmer wants to argue with

On May 21, 2004, the Supreme Court of Canada, in a 5-4 decision, found Saskatchewan farmer Percy Schmeiser guilty of violating the Monsanto Company's patented "Roundup-Ready" (RR) gene used in some canola seed. Documents from earlier court proceedings show that Monsanto ordered its investigators to trespass on Schmeiser's fields and collect samples from his crops as proof he was using their patented gene illegally. Schmeiser fought the case for seven years, arguing that the Monsanto-modified canola seeds landed on his farm by accident. Agriculture Canada scientists say wind can blow seeds or pollen between fields, meaning the DNA of crops in one field often mixes with that in another. Seeds or pollen can also be blown off trucks and farm equipment. Presumably, following this court decision, farmers not paying to use GMO seeds will be expected to locate any of these accidental plants in their fields and dig them up.

Sources: Grain.org; CBC News Online, "Percy Schmeiser's battle," May 21/04.

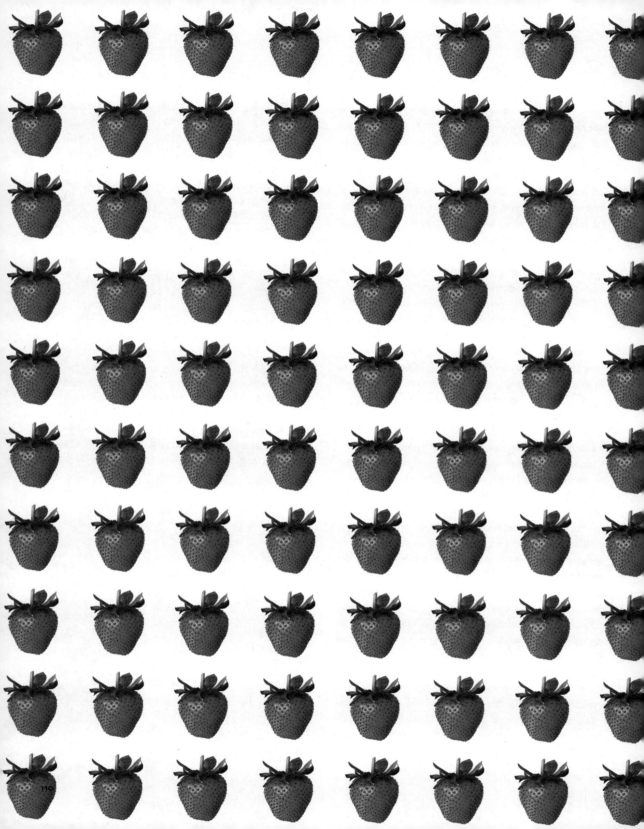

the factory farm across the road about who owns his crop, well they'll just see him in court.

Corn is just one example. For years, Monsanto and the others have been systematically buying up seed companies all over the world that sell seed for all the big commodity crops: corn, potatoes, soy, canola, wheat. They create their own patented varieties of these crops in the laboratory, then let the heirloom varieties slowly die out through cross-pollination and lack of replanting. It only takes a generation or so to lose an heirloom variety of a cultivated crop. Agricultural crops are not like weeds; they have been cultivated and nurtured by farmers for thousands of years to the point where they simply can't survive on their own—that's why you don't see vacant lots overgrown with corn, soy, or tomatoes. So if the agricultural community doesn't actively promote and support the heirloom varieties, they will disappear forever.

Ultimately, what you end up with is a monoculture—one variety that has been genetically modified and is pretty much genetically homogeneous from plant to plant. Now that might make it easier to make perfect apple pyramids in the grocery store, but it's just not how nature does things. What you lose with monoculture crops, along with common ownership, is the resiliency that comes from thousands of years of cross-pollination between related varieties and plants. So if you were to, say, introduce a disease into an area where all the corn plants are very similar genetically, that disease is likely to do much more damage than it would if there were numerous varieties planted and interspersed together, because some varieties might be less susceptible to the disease than others. Diversity is one way that nature ensures survival.

Then there is always the possibility that a genetically engineered trait placed in a food crop might find its way into a closely related plant that we might consider a weed. If Bt corn can be engineered to fight off the corn borer, what would happen if another plant, through cross-pollination, acquired the ability to resist the insects that keep it under control naturally? That's the problem when you start tampering with nature at the genetic level: once the genie is out of the bottle, it's not so easy to put it back in.

But I don't think the Monsantos of the world think in those terms. All they know is, if they can reduce the commodity crops down to just a few recognized varieties that they own, they can control the whole food chain—and to hell with the consequences. The farmers will go back to being serfs on the land, planting only those seeds that are allowed by the companies that own seed patents. Farmers who grow GE crops have to sign a contract with the seed company that says they can't plant seeds saved from their harvest for the next year because those seeds remain the property of the company. When they want to replant they have to renew their contract, and they can never break away because they can't guarantee none of the old seeds won't show up as plants in a new crop, free to cross-pollinate again.

It's an agricultural Catch-22, but that scenario is real, and it's happening right now, courtesy of genetic engineering. It may sound like science fiction to the average person, but it's absolute utopia for corporate agribusiness.

And honestly, what chance do traditional family farmers have against the money and influence of multinational corporations? Just like back when pesticides and herbicides came along, the independent farmer is often forced to plant GE seed, even if he or she doesn't want to, just to stay afloat. Small family farmers today usually have no control over their own seed stock; they are often in debt to some bank that has the right to "advise" them about what seed to plant; they can't protect their crops from cross-pollination; and they can't fight the agri-corps in court. It's a no-win situation for the traditional farmers all the way around. They can either sign on with the corporations or get pushed the hell out. That's why you see so many of the older farmers today selling up and moving off the land; they can't compete against the factory farms and they know it. But who do you think is right there waiting to scoop up these "unproductive," "unprofitable" family farms at auction?

And last, but certainly not least, there are the political implications of genetically modified food and corporate agriculture. In the United States, where the people are supposed to control the government, we've already allowed chemically treated, irradiated, and genetically modified food to take over our diet and almost wipe out

$24-million through soft money and individual donations; 7 of the 10 leading recipients of agri-corp donations in the House of Representatives sat on the Agricultural Committee that year. Ties between politicians and Big Agriculture have a huge influence on government policies in rural states as well. A 1999 survey in Virginia showed 29 of the 123 elected officials surveyed had an agricultural conflict of interest.
—KH.

Source: Williams, The Corruption of American Agriculture.

the inde-pendent farmer, but at least we have the option of saying "No." What happens in a developing country where the people have no control at all over their government and no way to voice their opposition?

Actually, the developing world is likely the next frontier for agribusiness. If we finally make enough noise in the developed world about all the negative shit that comes with genetic modification and corporate agriculture, they'll probably start moving their operations to Central America or Africa where they can just pay off government officials and run their business however they like, whether it's good or bad for people or for the environ-ment. The next Chernobyl may well come courtesy of biotechnology and corporate agriculture.

The biggest crock of all, of course, is when the big agri-corps try to convince us that genetic modification and corporate agriculture will allow us to conquer hunger around the world—as if they care. The fact is, we already produce far more food in the world than we could ever eat. I read one study that said we can pro-duce something like 4.5 pounds, or around 3,500 calo-ries, of food per person per day—not only enough to wipe out hunger but enough to make everyone fat. That's probably pretty accurate when you consider how much food we waste every day, especially in the devel-oped world. How much food do you think gets chucked

from the all-you-can-eat buffets across the country each day? Just think how much food you waste yourself in a day, or how much you eat and don't need.

So why is there so much hunger in the world? Why are there over thirty million people in the United States alone, the richest country in the world, who don't have enough to eat? It's not because we don't pro-duce enough food; it's because too many people don't make

enough money to buy food. It's because too much arable land is in the hands of too few people. These are the real issues, and screwing with the genetic code of a tomato isn't going to solve them. And even if genetic engi-neering made it possible for us to produce twice as much food as we do now, the developing world doesn't have the ability to distribute it or to store it. Besides, do you really think after spending so much time and money developing GE crops, the agri-corps are just going to give them away?

Big agribusiness loves to pull a little stunt called "poor washing." They say that the only people protest-ing against GE food are white, middle-class young peo-ple from wealthy countries, and they don't hear anyone complaining about it in places like India or Mexico or the Philippines. They say that a few activist college kids shouldn't be allowed to stand in the way of technology that has the potential to help millions, basically using the poverty and hunger of the developing world to stifle opposition and wash themselves clean. So what if they end up owning patents on every cash crop in the world? I guess that's beside the point. Make no mistake— genetically engineered food isn't about hunger; it's about greed.

It's probably not surprising that it was George Bush, Sr., who said it was OK for big agribusiness to go ahead with GE crop research in the first place. But then the Clinton administration basically ignored the issue. And Shrub Monkey, as I affectionately call him, sure as hell is not going to do anything about it now. Actually, politicians don't like to talk about things like genetically engineered food and corporate agriculture because they don't see them as partisan issues that will help them get elected. Most of them just try to avoid the subjects altogether.

The truth is, politicians from all parties take in big money from corporate agribusiness and the chemical industry. So you're not likely to see a politician looking to finance a re-election campaign in a rural state pushing some regulatory agency to do more research on genetically modified food, or to crack down on factory farms for screwing up the environment with their leeching pesticides or rivers of pig shit.

These corporations also spend a lot of money and effort trying to sell themselves to us. They spend millions of dollars every year in the *New York Times* and on National Public Radio so they can "inform the public" on the "wonders of biotechnology." ADM (a multinational food giant based in Illinois) likes to dress up a model from a Ralph Lauren ad in a denim jacket and put him on TV on Sunday morning during *Meet the Press* as a "typical family farmer" who is reaping the benefits of GE crops and modern farming methods. He's supposed to be just like you, just folks, a guy trying to make a living. The thing is, he doesn't look anything like the farmers you see in the newspapers auctioning off their farms.

It's all just noise, just spin. The agri-corps flood us with noise about improving nutrition, improving yields to fight hunger, improving the lives of farmers, just to try to divert our attention from what they're really up to. And as long as nobody asks any questions, that spin is all we have to go on.

At the end of the day, though, we have to ask ourselves if we really need to go down this road in the first place. Maybe we can clone sheep and alter the genetic code of a plant so it grows bigger, or has a nicer color or a nicer shape, but do we really need to? People in the scientific community often say to me, "Well, you can't stop technology." But is this a problem that needs a technological solution, or is it technology in search of a problem?

Oh yeah, let's not forget the sticky problem of ethics. You don't need to be religious to feel that it's somehow not ethically right to tamper with the very evolutionary essence of a living thing. Right now it's with plants and animals, but the potential is there to one day genetically engineer humans, so where do you draw the line? If it's all just about money, then there's no doubt there would be a huge demand for "designer" babies—"Just give us your details and we'll make 'em any way you want." But at least we know that's wrong. At least I hope we do.

We humans are simply curious by nature. We fiddle with things and change them around to see if they'll work better, and I understand that. Pushing the boundaries of science and technology has done wonderful things for humanity, but it's done plenty of shitty things too, and we need to make sure we know the difference before we forge ahead. It seems to me that pushing technology is fine when you're talking about toys like cell phones, computers, and satellites. But when it comes to my body, when it comes to what I put in my stomach and what I feed my children, that's when I want to slow down and think seriously about where technology is taking us.

The debate around genetic engineering and corporate agriculture generates a lot of noise, and I know at times the noise is deafening, like the sound of those crop dusters I tried to outrun on my bike on the SOL Tour. But the great thing is, you don't have to listen. You can shut off all that noise by doing one simple thing: reconnect with the planet. And you can do that by learning about the food you eat, where it comes from, and what happens to it before you put it in your body. You can do it by going to a farmers' market and buying organically produced food from people you know and trust. There are farmers out there who are hanging on and fighting to maintain an approach to food production they know is sustainable and right, and they need our support.

And after you get reconnected, you can use what you've learned to reconnect your family and friends. That's how we're going to take our food supply back—one stomach at a time, starting with yours.

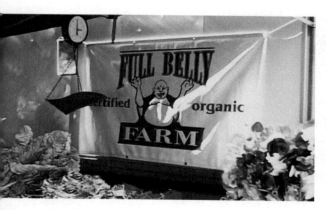

The Organic Solution

It sounds strange to me whenever I hear the media describe organic food and organic farming as some kind of fad, as if it was something some hippie farmers in California just dreamed up in the last few years. There is actually nothing new about organic food and organic farming; they've been around ever since we stepped out of the cave and picked some berries. It's just that they used to be known as "food" and "farming."

One hundred years ago all farming and all food was organic, at least according to today's definition of the word. But that all changed when the chemical companies figured they had a better way to grow plants and the agri-corporations decided you could apply the principles of the assembly line to the farmyard. When they were faced with these radical changes in their way of life, many

traditional farmers decided to sell off their farms to the corporations, rather than wait to go bankrupt trying to compete with them. As time passed and the specter of corporate agribusiness began to cast its shadow across the land, others gave in to the pressure and adopted the "modern" farming methods just to stay alive. Pretty soon the modern approach to farming, complete with its crop-dusted fields and force-fed livestock, became the standard. Today we see the result: what was natural is now unusual and the unnatural has become commonplace (children's hospitals, for example . . .).

Luckily for us though, traditional farming, or "organic" farming if you prefer, never really disappeared entirely. Organic food and organic farmers were always there, even if western society did forget about them for a while. In spite of all the pressure to conform over the years and decades, there were still farmers who rejected the chemicals and the corporate farming methods. Even before the scientists knew about the negative effects of pesticides and herbicides, many traditional farmers knew in their heart that it was the wrong approach. They could see what the chemicals did to the soil, wearing it out and robbing it of its natural ability to rejuvenate; they could see their livestock developing health problems that they'd never had before; and they could see the disastrous effect the harsh farm chemicals had on other plants and wildlife and the streams, ponds, and rivers. The strong ones decided they just couldn't accept that.

Organic farmers are a stubborn breed, that's for sure. They've managed to exist on the fringes of the agriculture industry for decades in spite of the best efforts of corporate agribusiness to wipe them out completely. To be an organic farmer means to make a conscious choice to go against the grain; if there are ninety-nine other farmers out there using chemicals on their crops, the organic farmer has to be willing to be the one who doesn't. He or she has to be the one who says no to bio-engineered seed, no to hormone-injected livestock, no to over-crowed barns and feeding pens. Every day it means having to stop, think, and then make that choice again. It's a real leap of faith, because there isn't some nationwide fast-food chain waiting to buy the crops or the livestock.

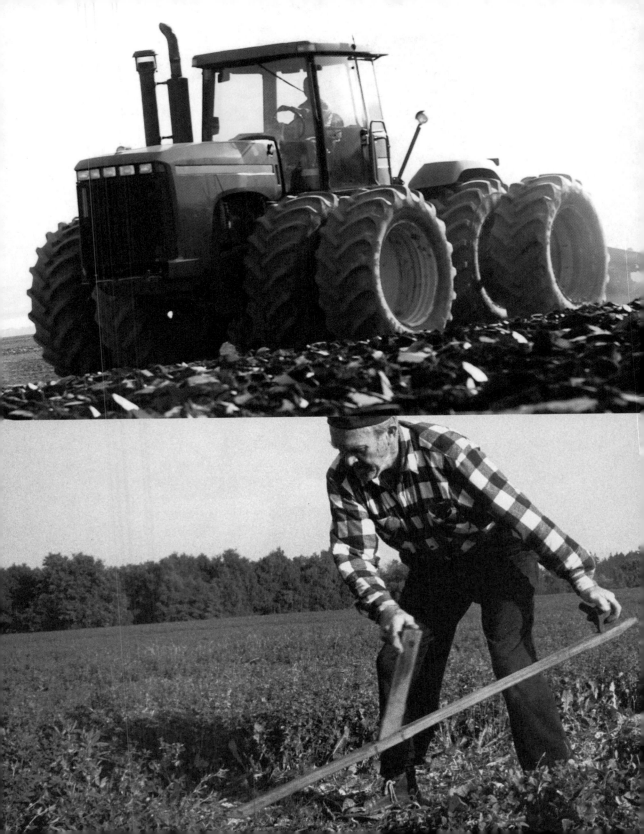

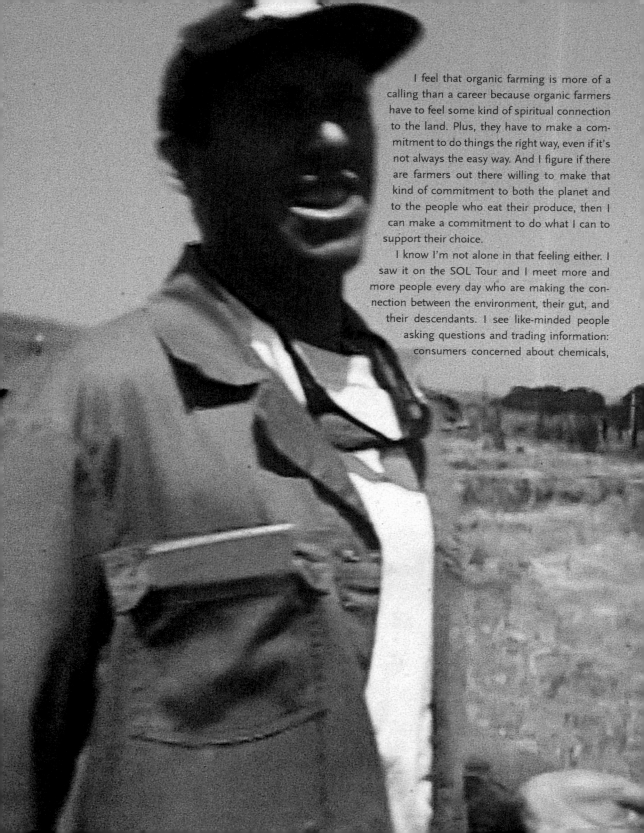

I feel that organic farming is more of a calling than a career because organic farmers have to feel some kind of spiritual connection to the land. Plus, they have to make a commitment to do things the right way, even if it's not always the easy way. And I figure if there are farmers out there willing to make that kind of commitment to both the planet and to the people who eat their produce, then I can make a commitment to do what I can to support their choice.

I know I'm not alone in that feeling either. I saw it on the SOL Tour and I meet more and more people every day who are making the connection between the environment, their gut, and their descendants. I see like-minded people asking questions and trading information: consumers concerned about chemicals, hormones, and synthetic genes in their food; small organic farmers trying to farm in a way that sustains both the land and themselves; and environmentalists fighting large corporations that see farming not as a way of life but as just another form of "resource extraction." These groups of people are building bridges that I believe will ultimately become the links in a worldwide organic food movement. And if we all get behind it, that movement has the potential to be just as strong and just as significant as the fight for civil rights in the 1960s, the struggle for the equality of women, or the anti-nuke movement.

Just like those other great struggles for positive change, the organic food movement has a lot of obstacles to overcome. Corporate agribusiness has way too much money invested in their chemicals, their factory farms, and their bio-tech research to ignore the threat posed by a strong organic food market. In fact, the battle has already begun on many fronts: you can see it in the way the agri-corps resist regulations that would require them to label chemically treated or genetically engineered food products; the way they are working to establish patents on the genetic codes of food crops and livestock; and the way they lobby the politicians to give them a free pass on our environment and a free hand with our food supply; and in the way they sue any organic farmers whose crops test positive for GE varieties they are not contracted to plant.

I've met a lot of people in my travels who are really discouraged about the current situation in agriculture, and they always ask me the same question: "How can the organic food movement hope to succeed against the money and political influence of these multinational corporations?" The answer, I believe, is to find their weakness and use it against them. The corporations may not care much about things like ethics, or morals, or fairness, but they do care about money. What the organic

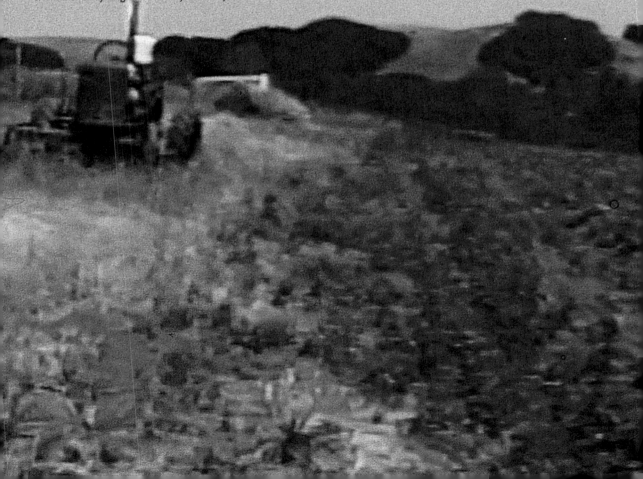

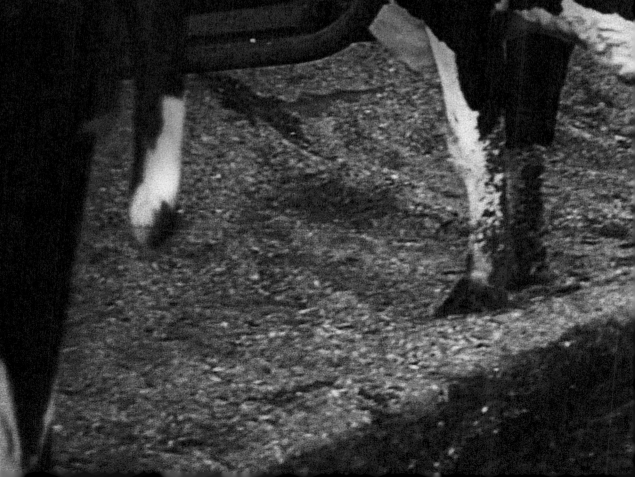

food movement needs to do if it's going to succeed in changing the world is become an economic force as well as a social one, and that's where the consumer can take control of this struggle. The chemical companies and the agri-corps may be able to control a lot of things but they can't control where you spend your money—at least not yet. Currently, the organic food market is growing by forty per cent a year. That's a hopeful sign.

Believe it or not, every time you resist the urge to spend your hard-earned money on some highly processed packaged food, you strike a blow for the organic food movement. And then if you ask the manager of your local grocery store why he doesn't stock organic products, you strike another blow. And if you actually take the time to go to your local farmers' market, meet the food producers there and build a relationship with them, and then lay your money down, well, that's the best protest you can make against corporate agribusiness.

I talk to people all the time about making the switch to organic, and most of the resistance I encounter centers on one thing: price. On the face of it, it's a pretty tough argument to counter; you can imagine some mother in the grocery store with the kids screaming and she sees "commercially grown" apples at 50 cents a pound and "organically grown" apples at $1.50 a pound. Obviously, the first thing she's going to think of is her pocketbook. But what I ask people to do is to try to see the bigger picture. While it is true that organically produced food usually costs more to buy than commercially produced food, that doesn't necessarily mean that the corporate stuff won't cost you more in the long run. It all depends on what you take into account when you calculate costs.

First of all, corporate food is cheaper to produce because the factory farm system was designed to make it that way. Factory farms fortify the soil with synthetic

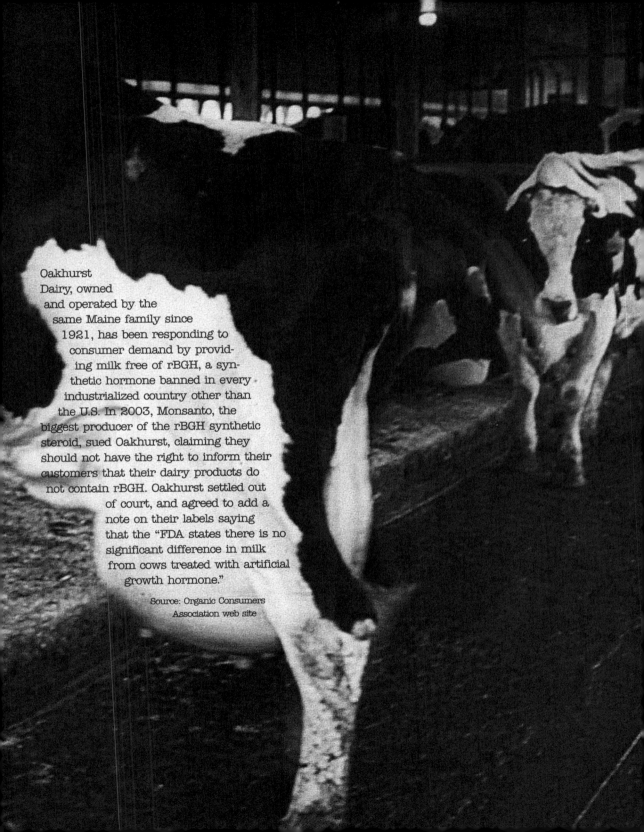

Oakhurst Dairy, owned and operated by the same Maine family since 1921, has been responding to consumer demand by providing milk free of rBGH, a synthetic hormone banned in every industrialized country other than the U.S. In 2003, Monsanto, the biggest producer of the rBGH synthetic steroid, sued Oakhurst, claiming they should not have the right to inform their customers that their dairy products do not contain rBGH. Oakhurst settled out of court, and agreed to add a note on their labels saying that the "FDA states there is no significant difference in milk from cows treated with artificial growth hormone."

Source: Organic Consumers Association web site

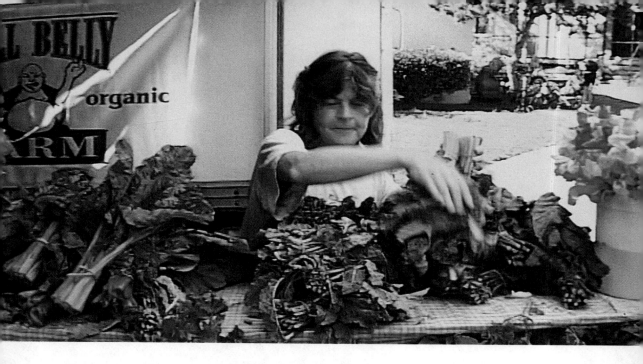

nutrients so they can pump more produce out of a smaller piece of land; they plant seeds that are genetically engineered to grow faster or fatter or with less water than normal seeds; and then they spray pesticides and herbicides to keep the insects and weeds from damaging even a tiny percentage of the crop. The result is a maximum yield of perfectly formed crops that they then harvest using as few workers as possible. Meanwhile, dairy cows are pumped full of hormones so they produce more milk, and cattle, pigs, and chickens are stuffed by the thousands into massive mechanized feeding pens while their untreated waste leeches into the streams and rivers.

The goal of all this chemical, biological and technological intervention is simple: to produce as much as possible as cheaply as possible. From a business perspective, the system works pretty well—for the agricorps and their shareholders. They're able to keep costs down and profit margins up, and most consumers don't care how something gets to the grocery store just as long as the price is right. But I don't think consumers would be nearly as happy with the corporate agriculture system if they thought for a minute about the price tag they don't see.

For example, one cost of corporate agriculture that doesn't get factored into the price is the cost to the environment. We're already paying millions of dollars in taxes to clean up the mess left in our waterways by chemical run-off from factory farms (as well as from mines, oil refineries, and so on), and what price can we put on the rivers, streams, and lakes that have been permanently damaged? You won't see that on your grocery bill, but you pay for it just the same.

I also believe if you were to compare a person on a corporate-food diet with someone eating a strictly organic diet you would find that there are more hidden costs associated with poorer health. Aside from the dangers of saturated fats and refined sugars, people who eat corporate food ingest far more chemicals and synthetic hormones than those who eat organic, and we still don't know what effect genetically modified food might have on our health down the road. So tack something on that corporate-food bill for bad health too.

Finally, there is the political cost of corporate agriculture. Forget the NRA—the chemical companies and the multinational food companies are some of the most powerful political lobbyists around. They provide campaign financing for politicians who make it possi-

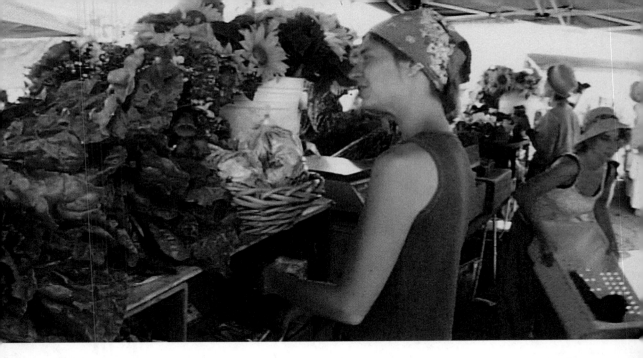

ble for them to do an end-run around environmental laws and food production regulations, and these same politicians funnel billions of tax dollars every year into huge farm subsidies. The politicians argue that the subsidies are needed to help family farmers stay on the land, but the truth is that we pay farm subsidies to keep prices stable so the agri-corps can guarantee good profit margins for their shareholders. So in reality, it doesn't really matter if you buy that corporate food at the grocery store or not, because you've already paid for it with your taxes anyway.

I think if average consumers take the time to add it all up, they'll see that eating organic really doesn't cost more than eating corporate; in the long run, it probably costs a lot less. Once you tack on the environmental cost, the health cost, and the political cost of corporate agriculture, there's really no comparison. In fact, I think it should piss people off that all those hidden costs aren't reflected in the price of commercially produced food at the grocery store. The fact is, cheap mass-produced food is a myth being perpetrated on the consumer by corporate agribusiness, with the willing assistance of its political appointees. I believe it's high time we exploded that myth and pulled the cur-

tain back on corporate agriculture once and for all.

If you still feel organic food is too expensive, then ask yourself why it costs as much as it does. The most obvious reason, of course, is that organic farmers don't use all the chemical and technological tricks that allow the factory farms to boost production and cut costs. That means the organic farmer takes more time to let things grow and develop naturally—working *with* the land, not just *on* the land. And because they refuse to screw with the natural balance in the ecosystem, they risk losing a bigger percentage of their crop to insects and competing plants, but it's a risk they're willing to take. Finally, by definition, organic farming is about people working with the land, therefore it's far more labor-intensive (but God forbid we should actually create jobs in agriculture).

In the end, organic yields tend to be smaller but the quality is infinitely better. So given all the time and effort that goes into the creation of organic food, I think consumers should be happy to spend a little more for a premium product that tastes better, doesn't have any weird shit on it or in it, doesn't harm the environment, and helps preserve a way of life that has served humanity well for thousands of years.

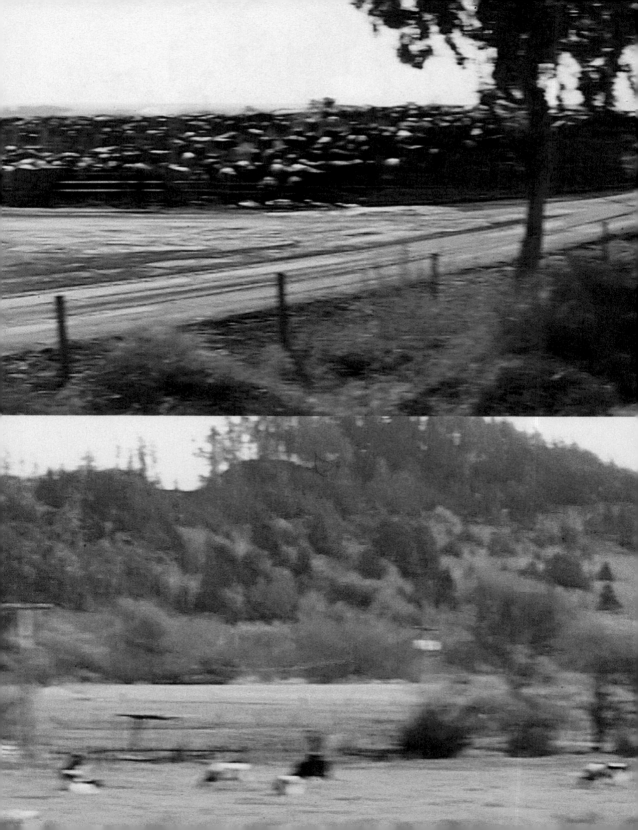

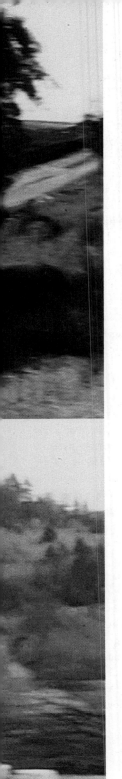

As if that wasn't enough, there is something else to consider when you compare prices for organic and corporate food. On top of all the normal costs of production, the organic farmer also has to meet a burden of proof that corporate agribusiness does not. If organic farmers want get the most out of their decision to do things the right way, they have to pay some kind of third-party certification organization to come in and evaluate their operation and farming methods and then give them the "organic" seal of approval. Then, in order to take advantage of that distinction and to differentiate their products from those of their corporate competitors, they have to invest in labeling that makes it clear their product is, in fact, organic. Certification is a big part of the cost of organic food but, once again, it's worth it for the consumer because it buys peace of mind.

It's a totally messed-up system when you think about it: organic farmers have to pay money because they go out of their way not to poison the earth, air, water, and everything living on it or in it, while factory farms get subsidies for doing exactly that.

One of the most irritating things for me about the whole corporate agriculture system is that the corporations are so smug about what they do, as if they're doing humanity some great service by inventing bionic corn. In fact, lots of the people involved in corporate agriculture don't see what they do as being much different from what organic farmers do. They figure all agriculture, whether it's traditional or modern, is a manipulation of nature, so what's the big deal about giving farmers new tools, like chemicals and bio-engineered seed, to help make that manipulation more efficient?

Well, I'm not denying that human beings have manipulated nature in numerous ways over the centuries in order to ensure their survival—from the domestication of the cow to the development of the modern corn plant. The thing is, those changes always came at a pace that nature could handle, over hundreds, even thousands, of years. That's not the case anymore. With modern chemicals, machinery, and especially biotechnology, the human race now has the power to alter thousands of years of evolution in an instant. We can wipe out old plant and animal species and introduce new ones on a whim. Evolution just doesn't work that fast, and I believe it's not supposed to.

I guess that's the bottom line for me when it comes to choosing organic: I just know in my heart that the organic approach is the right approach. And if "right" is too strong a word for you, how about "proper"? I think it's proper to have a farm that mimics nature, with different kinds of plants growing side by side in the same field, attracting all kinds of pollinators and predators in a balanced, interdependent ecosystem, rather than rows and rows of one crop in a totally unnatural monoculture. I think it's proper to let livestock roam freely around the farm, foraging on grass and weeds and dropping their organic fertilizer in neat piles on the ground, rather than force-feeding hormone-laced feed to them in overcrowded barns. I think it's proper to have lots of people working small family farms, as opposed to having a few corporations running huge factory farms. And I think it's proper to save the heirloom varieties of food crops that have been stewarded down through the centuries by our ancestors and handed down to us by our grandma and grandpa to be shared by farmers everywhere, instead of allowing the Monsantos of the world to put a patent on every living thing. If that's not right, I'd like to know what is.

You know, in the industrialized world, especially in the United States, we pray at the altar of the almighty dollar. I know we live in a democracy, but your real voting power is in your wallet, and every time you enter the grocery store you have a chance to make a statement about where you think the real public interest lies. I always ask people to remember that when you buy organic, you're not just doing the right thing for your body; you're making an investment in the future and a statement about the kind of planet you want your children to inherit.

And no matter how insignificant you might feel when you make that statement, you should never doubt that the big corporations can hear you when you buy organic. Because when your dollars are added to all the others, the organic food market grows a little bit more and trims just a little bit more off corporate agribusiness's bottom line. Most people eat at least three times a day, so that's at least three chances every day to have a positive influence, to rebuild your body with something righteous, something good, something that's going to support the planet.

If enough people start taking their dollars out of the corporate loop, it won't be long before those dogs start to follow the money. At some point, it'll start making financial sense for the agri-corps to actually convert corporate operations back to organic. As consumers, we can push that change by demanding organic alternatives at the grocery store and in restaurants; just look how quickly the industry responded with low-fat and low-carbohydrate products when more and more people finally got tired of being fat.

Once the industry starts to change, the politicians won't be far behind. When you think about it, changing your diet is like entering the ground floor of social activism.

I believe there are more than enough positive reasons for anyone to make the switch to an organic diet, but if eating better-tasting, more nutritious food that doesn't harm the planet isn't enough for you, you might consider this: It is a simple fact that there are about twice as many people on the earth today as there were the day I was born a little more than four decades ago. And if I manage to live to twice my current age, that number will double again, meaning there will be four times as many people on the earth when I die as there was when I was born.

On top of that, consider the fact that seventy-five percent of the topsoil—the fertile earth needed to grow things—that was in North America when the pilgrims arrived 400 years ago is now gone. It takes something like 500 years to produce one inch of topsoil, and we've already lost three quarters of what we had. It's no coincidence that most of that soil erosion has taken place only in the last hundred years, when modern farm machinery and chemicals came on the scene.

In light of these two simple facts, you don't have to be a biotech engineer to see that we are on a path right now that simply is not sustainable. Our population is growing while the raw material we used to feed that population, the soil, is drying up and blowing away. We're wearing out our planet, and for what? Cheap vegetables? Bug-proof corn? Chicken McNuggets?

Remember, every great civilization that has ever flourished on the planet Earth has always failed for one reason: they couldn't provide for their own people. We have allowed corporate agribusiness to take over the task of providing for our society, and it is in the process of burning up our agricultural resources for the sake of quick corporate profits. I believe if we continue down the road we're currently traveling, it will eventually lead to a crisis in the food supply—if not in our lifetime, then in the lifetime of our children, or our children's children.

It's time to wake up. We're in the same position the dinosaurs were in, except they didn't know they were marching toward extinction. We should. The good news is we have a way out; we have a ready alternative if we just choose to take it. An organic revolution, based on sustainable agriculture in tune with nature, has the power to save our bodies, our communities, and our planet. You can be a part of that revolution, starting with the next dollar you lay down.

100% Organic
c o t t o n

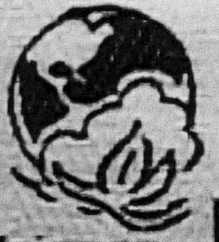

made in u.s.a.

L

Beneficial T's ®

Shirt

MAD COWBOY

Howard Lyman

My name is Howard Lyman and I am a fourth-generation farmer, rancher, and feed lot operator from Montana. At least that's what I used to do; today I have a different job. Today I spend about eleven out of twelve months a year traveling around the world—probably 100,000 miles a year—talking to people about the amount of animal products people should have in their diet, which, you may be surprised to hear, is none.

Now, I know coming from a person like me that might sound strange. After all, I am an ex-cattleman, one that at one time had 7,000 head of cattle, along with 12,000 acres of poison crops and thirty employees to look after it all. But today I eat no animal products at all; I don't eat 'em and I don't wear 'em. I am strictly vegan, and the produce I eat is 100 per cent organic. I'm a changed person. It was a change I had to make, and a change I believe we all have to make for the good of the planet. Because I can tell you, as somebody who spent the better part of his lifetime—forty-five years—in the animal production business, what we are doing today in North America in terms of food production is absolutely, totally unsustainable.

My wake-up call came in 1979. Back then, I guess you could say I was about as big a success story as you can be as rancher and farmer. I loved it too—I had twenty tractors and thirty trucks and three or four combines at $100,000 a piece, and when I got to the point where I could write a check for one million dollars and it didn't bounce, I felt like I was the Donald Trump of the agriculture business.

Then I started having problems with my back. First I couldn't get out of bed in the morning, then I started having trouble walking and getting up and down stairs. My condition got worse and worse, until I finally ended up in the hospital, paralyzed from the waist down.

The doctors did their tests and broke the news that I had a tumor on my spinal cord that was affecting the mobility of my legs. They told me that if the tumor was on the outside of the

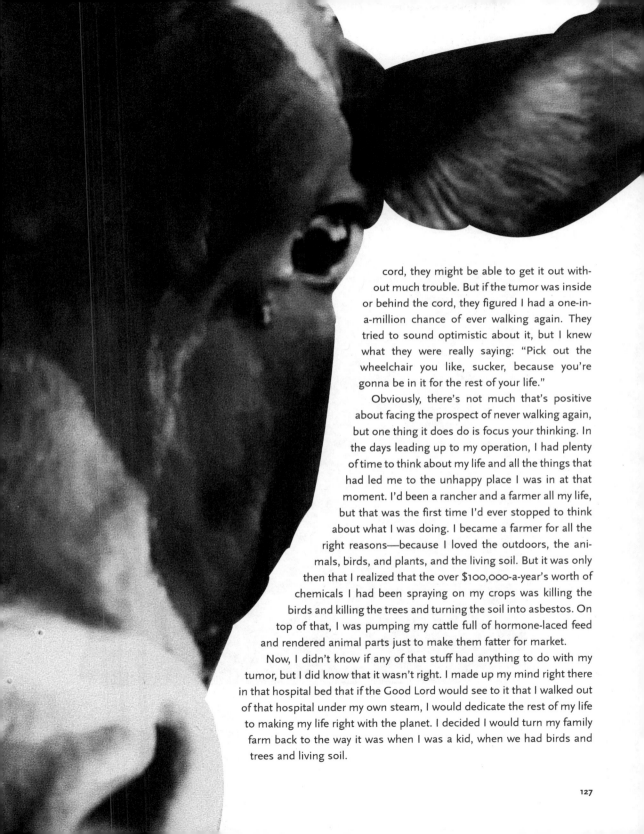

cord, they might be able to get it out without much trouble. But if the tumor was inside or behind the cord, they figured I had a one-in-a-million chance of ever walking again. They tried to sound optimistic about it, but I knew what they were really saying: "Pick out the wheelchair you like, sucker, because you're gonna be in it for the rest of your life."

Obviously, there's not much that's positive about facing the prospect of never walking again, but one thing it does do is focus your thinking. In the days leading up to my operation, I had plenty of time to think about my life and all the things that had led me to the unhappy place I was in at that moment. I'd been a rancher and a farmer all my life, but that was the first time I'd ever stopped to think about what I was doing. I became a farmer for all the right reasons—because I loved the outdoors, the animals, birds, and plants, and the living soil. But it was only then that I realized that the over $100,000-a-year's worth of chemicals I had been spraying on my crops was killing the birds and killing the trees and turning the soil into asbestos. On top of that, I was pumping my cattle full of hormone-laced feed and rendered animal parts just to make them fatter for market.

Now, I didn't know if any of that stuff had anything to do with my tumor, but I did know that it wasn't right. I made up my mind right there in that hospital bed that if the Good Lord would see to it that I walked out of that hospital under my own steam, I would dedicate the rest of my life to making my life right with the planet. I decided I would turn my family farm back to the way it was when I was a kid, when we had birds and trees and living soil.

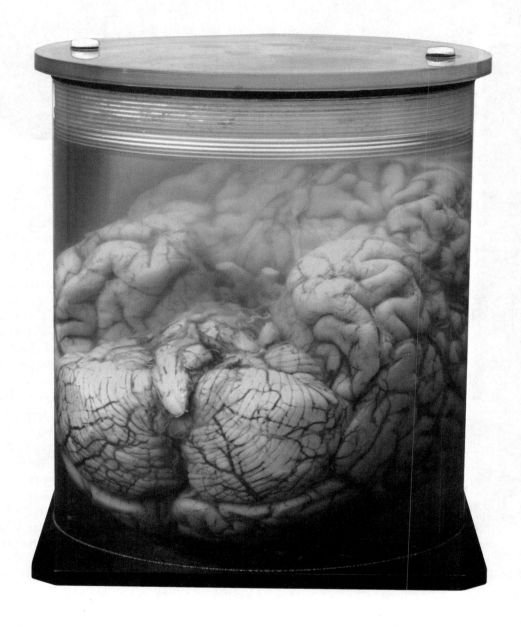

The doctors operated on me for twelve hours. Sure enough, the tumor was under my spinal cord, and the doctors were afraid to lift the cord to get at it. All they could do was pick a nerve they thought the tumor was attached to and cut it and hope they could pull it out like a fish on a line. So they picked one, cut it, and pulled out a tumor the size of my thumb. I walked out of that hospital on my own two feet—a one-in-a-million shot. Now, I don't think I walked away from that operation just because of the skill of those surgeons, and I don't think I walked away because of the care I received in the hospital. I think I walked out by the grace of God because of the promise that I made, and I've spent every day since then living up to that promise.

Back in the early 1990s, I started to talk to people about a condition that I'd seen from time to time in cattle over the years called bovine spongiform encephalopathy, or BSE. Well, today everybody knows about Mad Cow Disease, but back then when I first started talking about the danger it posed to humans, people told me I had holes in my brain. People aren't laughing about Mad Cow anymore, and today I find that the same people who wouldn't listen a decade ago are suddenly very eager to hear about just how much trouble I think we're in with this.

Back when I started to really research BSE, scientists were still struggling to figure out exactly what it was. It was a pretty rare thing up until the mid-1980s, when it started to show up with startling regularity in cattle in England. They knew that it was some kind of invasive pathogen that somehow got into a cow's nervous system and began to slowly eat away at its brain tissue, causing it to shake and stagger, before ultimately killing the animal. What they didn't know was what kind of pathogen it was or how it got into the cow in the first place. The penny dropped when they realized that BSE looked a lot like a brain-wasting condition in sheep called "scrapie," and British farmers had been feeding rendered sheep carcasses to cattle for years.

Once the scientists knew the source of the condition, they had to isolate the pathogen and figure out how to kill it. First they thought it was a slow-growing virus or bacterium, which would have made treating it relatively easy. But after experimenting on it they found it could routinely survive temperatures of 340 degrees centigrade (almost 650 degrees Fahrenheit), plus it had no RNA or DNA, which means it couldn't be a virus or bacterium. Finally they decided that it was a prion, which is another word for an abnormal protein. Under a microscope, a normal protein has a kind of spiral shape, but the protein that causes Mad Cow is long and flat. Now, the problem with a protein is that it's not a living thing; you can't kill it with temperature, you can't kill it with chemical solvents, and you can't kill it with radiation. The truth is, there is nothing in this world that we know of that can deactivate an abnormal protein. In fact, the only way to avoid the effects of pathogens like BSE is not to ingest them in the first place.

So the Brits stopped feeding sheep to cows in 1989, and they figured they had BSE under control—at least they thought they did, until 1996. In 1996, British doctors noticed a striking similarity between the Swiss-cheese brains of cows that had died of BSE and the brains of ten humans who had died of a rare brain-wasting condition called Creutzfeldt-Jakob Disease (CJD). The doctors believed that the pathogen had jumped the species barrier for the second time—first from sheep to cows, then from cows to humans. Well, once British consumers put two and two together, the writing was on the wall for the British beef industry. The only thing they could do to restore public confidence in British beef was to start fresh with a new BSE-free herd, so that's just what they did. More than four million head of cattle worth 7.5-billion dollars were slaughtered, incinerated, and plowed under in a matter of months.

Naturally, when consumers in countries all over the world saw what was going on in Britain, they started to ask questions about the beef in their own country. Of course, the respective beef industries in every country around the world were quick to stand up and say loudly, "We don't have Mad Cow in our herd; it's just those folks over in England that have it." That is what they said in France and Germany, although they had had cases of CJD in those countries.

That's what the beef industry in the United States said as well, but I knew damn well they couldn't say for sure that the U.S. cattle herd was completely BSE-free. Ranchers were still feeding rendered cow carcasses to cattle in the U.S. in 1996, just as they had done for years. I knew because I'd done it myself. So knowing how abnormal proteins work, and knowing that an abnormal protein causes BSE, what were we doing with cattle in North America? We were pumping them full of protein—maybe normal, maybe abnormal—in the form of rendered animal feed to make them fat for slaughter. We were feeding cows to cows, and likely producing more and more of the stuff we know we can't kill in the process.

So I started to speak out on the issue, telling people the truth about BSE and the truth about how the cattle industry in the U.S. really operated. With everything going on in England, the Mad Cow scare was big news, and it wasn't long before I got a call to appear on the *Oprah Winfrey Show* to talk about it. I was invited to appear along with Dr. Gary Weber from the National Cattlemen's Beef Association, an organization I was once a part of, and one that didn't like me very much anymore.

The show aired in April 1996. Oprah started off by asking me to explain why I felt Mad Cow had the potential to make AIDS look like the common cold. I explained how cows that get sick or die before they can be slaughtered, called "downers" in the industry, are routinely ground up into feed and fed back to other cows. So if even one of these downer cows has BSE, it has the potential to infect thousands of other cows through the feed chain.

Oprah looked at the guy from the Cattlemen's Association and asked him straight: "Are we feeding cattle to the cattle?"

I'll never forget what he said. He kind of squirmed in his chair and cleared his throat and finally said, "There is a limited amount of that done in the United States."

That statement almost floored me. As a former cattle rancher and feed lot owner, I knew for a fact that probably ninety-five percent of all the cattle fed in factory feed lots at that time were eating the remains of animals, and not just the remains of other cows. But that wasn't the most amazing statement made on the show.

At one point, Oprah looked kind of sick to her stomach, then she uttered a statement that would come back

to haunt both of us: "It has just stopped me cold from eating another burger."

Now Oprah didn't say, "I think U.S. meat is infected with BSE." She didn't say to her twenty million viewers, "You should stop eating meat." All she said was that hearing the truth about the U.S. beef industry was making her think twice about her diet. And for that, she got both of us sued.

A few days after the show, I got a call from a writer from a national news magazine who asked me, "By the way, do you realize you're being sued by the Cattlemen's Association, along with Oprah Winfrey and Harpo Productions?" I called the Oprah show right away and, sure enough, the Cattlemen were after both of us for "spreading misconceptions about U.S. beef."

Now, I'm not saying I wasn't worried at all about the suit but I do have a Doctor of Laws degree, so I know a thing or two about the law. The first law is, you never sue anyone who has nothing—which is me. The second law is, you never sue anyone who talks to twenty million people every day. That is Oprah Winfrey.

Well, believe it or not, we finally ended up in court two years later in Amarillo, Texas. The Cattlemen's Association had insisted on going ahead with the lawsuit, even though, in 1997, the USDA (United States Department of Agriculture) and the FDA (Food and Drug Administration) had done exactly what I called for on the show: they passed a regulation that prohibited the feeding of rendered ruminants to other ruminants (a ruminant being a cud-chewing animal, like a cow, sheep, or goat). Given that, I figured we'd get down there and the judge would dismiss the whole thing; I was wrong.

I wasn't in Amarillo very long before it started to hit home that I was right in the very heart of Texas beef country. As a matter of fact, some twenty-five per cent of all the cattle feed produced in the U.S. comes from the Amarillo area. There are 120 feedlots with an average of about 55,000 head of cattle each surrounding the city, and the largest single employer is a slaughter facility. When I saw a bumper sticker that said, "The only Mad Cow in Texas is Oprah," I knew we were in trouble.

We showed up at the courthouse for the first day of the trial and the place was just crawling with media and

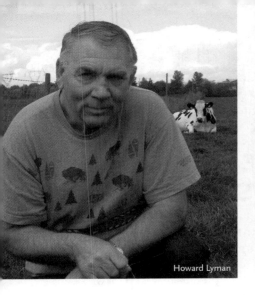
Howard Lyman

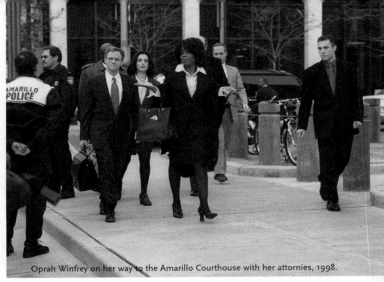
Oprah Winfrey on her way to the Amarillo Courthouse with her attornies, 1998.

local people who worked in the beef industry shouting insults at us. Obviously, the first thing my lawyer did was ask the judge, a little seventy-two-year-old lady, for a change of venue. But that old bird was tough, and she just slammed that mallet down on the bench and said, "Motion denied." Then they brought in the jury pool — about 140 people, and you never saw so many cowboy hats, cowboy boots and big belt buckles in your life.

By the time the trial got started, my backside was so puckered up I could barely sit down. Oprah was running scared too at the beginning, but once Dr. Phil started working on her, her whole attitude changed. She brought her whole show down to Amarillo and turned the national spotlight on the city, and I believe the pressure started working on the jury; in their hearts they knew that we hadn't done anything but tell the truth, and they didn't want to make Amarillo look like some cowboy backwater town. In the end, a jury that was absolutely steeped in cattle culture found that we were not liable.

Of course, the Cattlemen's Association couldn't let it go at that. They appealed the decision to the Fifth Circuit Court of Appeals and a year later we got a unanimous verdict from that court that everything I said on the *Oprah Winfrey Show* was true and the truth was not actionable. The Cattlemen didn't like that either, so they applied for a re-hearing of the case. The Fifth Circuit Court denied it. Then a bunch of other cattle ranchers went forty miles up the road to Dumas, Texas, and filed

exactly the same cause of action in state court. Not being from Texas, I applied to have the case moved to federal court, and they appealed that.

Given that a representative of the beef industry admitted on Oprah's program in 1996 that they were, in fact, feeding cows to cows at that time, you have to ask yourself why they just can't seem to face the truth that came out on that show. Since 1998, the cattle industry has been arguing over something the Fifth Circuit Court of Appeals ruled was "not actionable" years ago. For Oprah and me, this case was about freedom of speech, about my right to voice the truth and her right to express her opinion. But it was never about that for the beef industry. For them it was about the golden rule: "If you have enough gold, you should be entitled to make the rules."

The saddest thing is, for the beef industry, the potential impact of BSE on humans isn't a health issue, it's a public relations issue. For me though, BSE or Mad Cow or CJD or whatever you want to call it is an opportunity to make people actually think about what they are eating. It's sad, but it took people dying of a terrible brain-wasting disease to start people asking where their meat comes from and how it is processed. And now that we are asking those questions, we have a chance of heading off a worldwide epidemic.

The beef industry says it stopped feeding cows to cows in 1997, but that doesn't mean the problem is solved. It only takes an amount of material the size of a peppercorn to infect a human with BSE. And from the time that a human is infected, it can take anywhere from ten to forty years before they show any symptoms. When the symptoms do show up, you live maybe six to eighteen agonizing months, and every person that is infected will die.

On the Oprah show, Dr. Weber said that the beef industry has scientific proof that BSE doesn't exist in the United States. But the truth is, we slaughter about thirty-six million head of cattle a year in the U.S. And out of that thirty-six million head, we only test about 2,300 for BSE, which is about half of one per cent. In Switzerland they test 1.75 per cent of all slaughtered cattle for BSE. If we were to do the same thing in the United States, we would be looking at the brains of about 630,000 animals, instead of 2,700. In Japan they test the brain of every single cow that goes to slaughter.

There is a good reason why we only test 2,700 slaughtered cows in the U.S. every year for BSE. The rea-son is we have a system here that works on the principle of "Don't look; don't find." We are also using testing methods that can't detect whether or not an animal had BSE if it has been dead for twenty-four hours. And we use a test that takes ten days to complete, even though there are other testing methods that have been developed in other countries that can produce a result within five hours.

Why can't we tell the American people the truth about this stuff? Because there is too much money in the cattle business, that's why. There could be millions of consumers at risk in the United States but we are unwilling to really determine the extent of the problem because the government doesn't want to upset the beef industry. And if you don't believe that's true, try saying you don't want to eat hamburgers on national television and see what happens.

Howard Lyman is the author of Mad Cowboy: Plain Truth from the Cattle Rancher Who Won't Eat Meat *(Scribner, 1998). His website is www.madcowboy.com.*

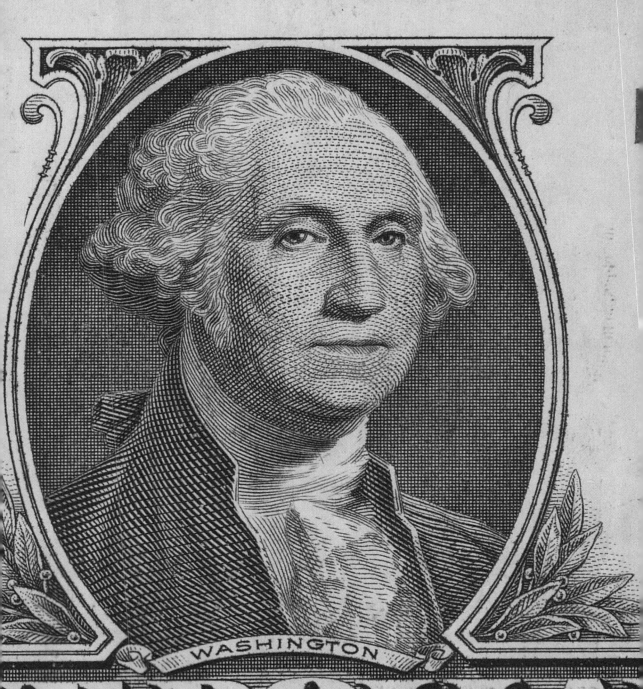

WASHINGTON

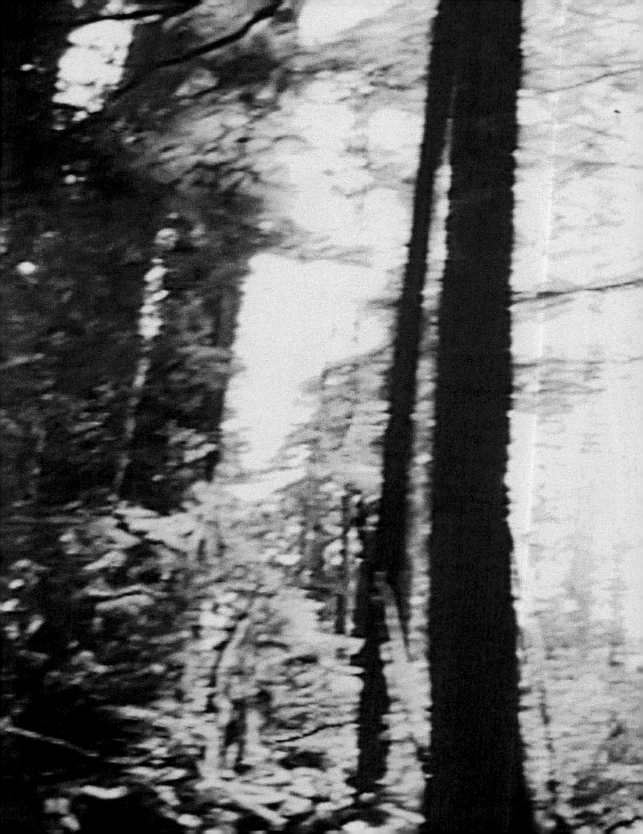

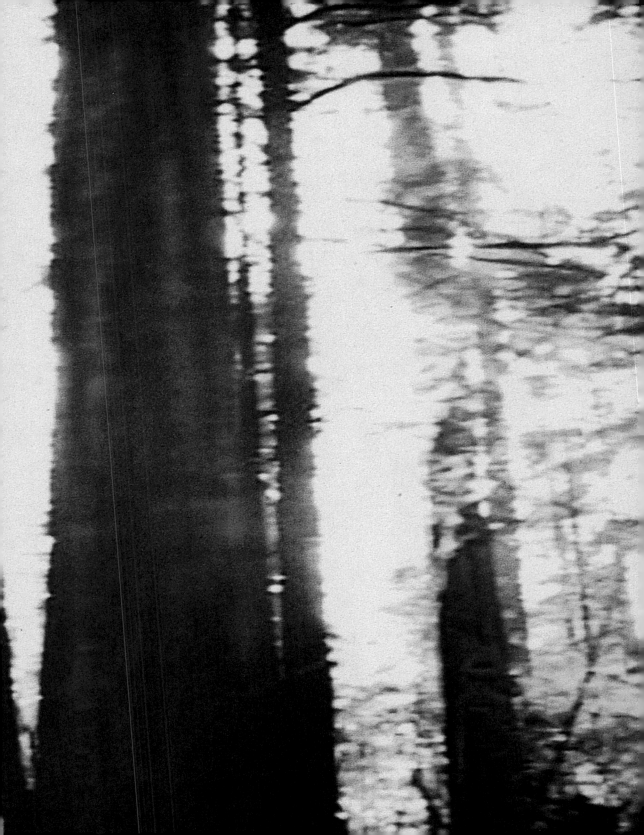

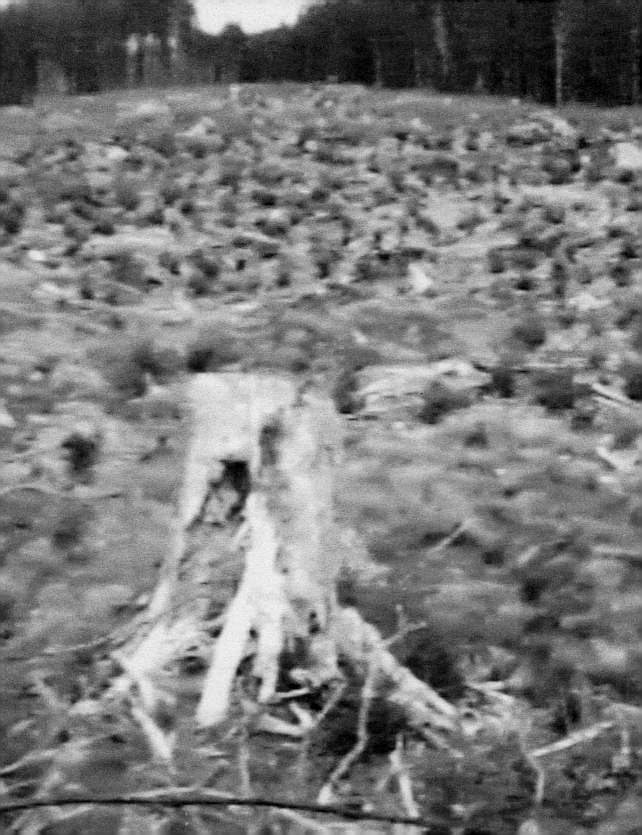

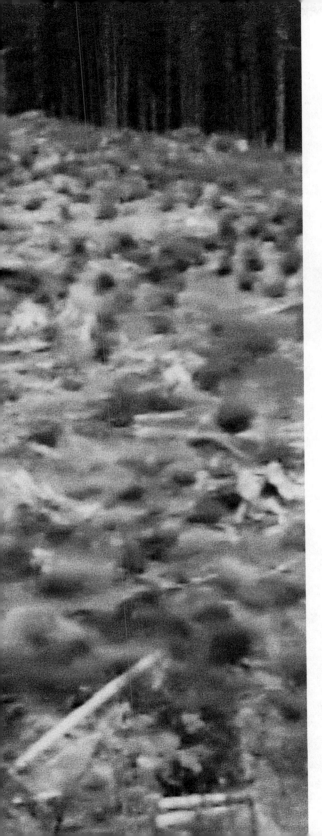

WOOD AND PAPER

As the SOL Tour began to wind its way down the West Coast into southern Washington State and Oregon, we started to see lots of trucks on the highway hauling huge logs to the paper mills. These were big mature trees that had probably stood for centuries before the white man ever set foot in the Pacific Northwest, and here they were dead, stretched out on the bed of a tractor trailer and destined to become pages in the financial section of the *Wall Street Journal*.

The trucks all had a sign on the back that read: "Warning: Logs can kill." That always struck me as more than a little ironic; I wonder what kind of sign the trees would put up to warn other trees about the danger of humans.

Another sign I saw along the way was more sad than ironic. It read, "America's First Tree Farm," and it stood on the edge of acres of neatly planted rows of trees that were all the same height. The sign was put there by Weyerhaeuser, one of the largest lumber companies in the world, and they were obviously really proud of all the work they were doing to "sustain our forest resources for the future." That's a point of view I could never wrap my head around; it was like they were saying, "Well yeah, we did cut down acres and acres of old-growth forest, but now we've got this great tree farm, so it's cool." Well, if you ask me, it's not cool.

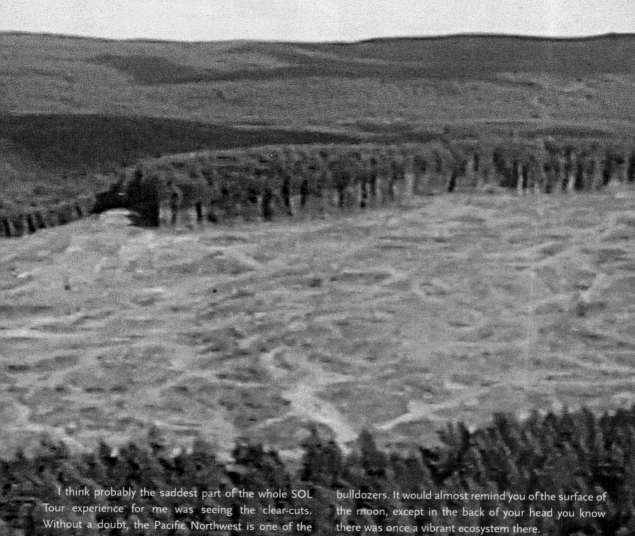

I think probably the saddest part of the whole SOL Tour experience for me was seeing the clear-cuts. Without a doubt, the Pacific Northwest is one of the most beautiful parts of North America: It's lush, sunny, warm, moist, green—it's like, every possible spot where something could grow has got some kind of plant on it. And then you hit the clear-cuts. A clear-cut is like an open wound in the landscape that comes out of nowhere and seems to go for miles. Not only are all the trees gone, big ones and small ones, the landscape itself is devastated, ground up and plowed under by bulldozers. It would almost remind you of the surface of the moon, except in the back of your head you know there was once a vibrant ecosystem there.

The goal of the clear-cut method of "tree harvesting" is total devastation—they cut it, burn the undergrowth, then spray it with Agent Orange or some other poison so any living plant there is wiped out. That paves the way for them to plant their little tree farm in nice neat rows where there are no other plants competing with the cash crop for sun and moisture. It's nothing more than a tree factory really—no diversity of plants, birds, and animals;

just young trees planted so they can be cut down again. I thought to myself as I rode past, "Man, if that's the future of our forest resources, there is no future."

Anyone who's ever walked through an old-growth forest knows what a joke it is when the paper and lumber companies say, "We're the model of sustainability because we plant two trees for every one we cut down." The problem is it's not just about the trees, and that's something the logging companies just don't want to admit; it's about whole ecosystems that take hundreds, even thousands, of years to create.

If you want to be honest about it, an old-growth forest and a tree farm have nothing in common except that they both have trees. A natural forest has a diversity of tree and plant species with plants of different ages. It's survival of the fittest—the trees and plants that have the best access to light and moisture grow the biggest and live the longest, while the ones that don't survive fall to the forest floor and decompose, putting minerals and nutrients back into the soil and offering shelter for insects and small animals. When the trees get really big, like in a true old-growth forest, there are only about forty or fifty trees growing per acre. The leaf canopy blocks out the sun and creates a kind of magical open space below. Larger animals like deer and elk can move easily through the trees; owls, hawks, and eagles can fly through the big spaces hunting for mice and rabbits. In some places in California, although there aren't many left, there are massive trees that are 300 feet tall and maybe a thousand years old. I can tell you, when you're standing on the forest floor under the big trees like that, it's like you're in a kind of natural cathedral that's as breathtaking as any man-made one in Europe.

A man-made tree farm, or tree factory, on the other

hand, doesn't look like anything Mother Nature would ever create. Usually it's one species of tree, planted all at the same time in rows at a density of about two or three hundred trees per acre. When the trees grow that close together, the branches tend to intertwine, making it impossible for large animals to walk through. So the deer and the elk get forced out into the open fields, where they piss off the farmers, and out onto the highway, where they get hit by trucks. Plus, the cover becomes so dense that the predatory birds can't fly through it and they can't even see the damn ground to hunt. And if a tree falls for some reason, it gets cut up and hauled the hell out of there right away so it doesn't get in the way when it's time to bring the mechanical tree-cutter through again.

I guess if you had to sum up all the differences between an old-growth forest and a tree farm in one word, it would be *sustainability*. A natural forest is designed by nature to be a sustainable ecosystem, where diverse plant and animal species work together to help each other survive. A tree farm is only designed to sustain its cash crop, a single species of tree, and only until it's profitable to cut it down.

See, the logging companies are only interested in maximizing the number of board feet of lumber or the amount of wood pulp they can extract from a given acre of property in a given amount of time. They might work on a twenty-year cycle in a certain area, where they clear-cut the old growth, replant, then come back in twenty years to do it all over again. We passed thousands of acres that had either been recently clear-cut or clear-cut ten or fifteen years ago and replanted, only to be clear-cut again. At that rate, those forests have no chance of ever returning to a state that resembles the way they were originally.

The problem is, nature prefers something closer to a 300-year growth cycle; actually, I think they would prefer, like us, to live out their natural lifespan. But that timetable just doesn't work for our paper-hungry society. When the personal computer came along, all the experts were saying it would cut way down on the amount of paper people use—"the paperless society," anybody remember that? If anything, we use more paper today than we did before we had computers; according to the Sierra Club, paper consumption in the U.S. grew by 44 pounds (20 kilograms) per capita between 1992 and 1997. Today, half the trees cut down in the United States every year are cut down to make paper products that are either thrown away after one use or not used at all.

Nature's 300-year growth cycle obviously doesn't work for the big corporations that cut down the trees and provide us with our paper and lumber. They can make a lot more money a hell of a lot faster by clear-cutting a whole forest and processing all the trees at once than they can by cutting trees down selectively over time. And the people who run those companies and who own their shares won't be around to see the fallout in 300 years, so they don't give a damn; hell, lots of them'll be dead in twenty years. They want as much profit as they can get from those "forest resources" right now. They're in the logging business, after all, not in the business of maintaining ecosystems. Just ask 'em.

Another thing the big logging corporations don't give a damn about is the people who live and work in the logging communities, and we met a lot of them on our ride. I don't have a problem with the loggers themselves or the people who work in the lumber and paper mills. I may not agree with what the industry they work in is doing, but that doesn't mean I don't respect them. They're hardworking people like anybody else, trying to live where they want to live and provide for their families. And I also understand that for many people in those communities, logging has been in their family for generations. For them, the forest industry isn't just a job, it's a way of life.

For the most part, we got a good reception from people we met along the way in the logging communities, but there were quite a few people who didn't like what we were doing one bit. There were times when I could feel a real hatred coming from people; they'd yell at us as we rode past, "Hey Woody Allen, we don't like tree-huggers around here."

One group of angry people I met told me that the local paper mill got shut down and a whole bunch of people got thrown out of work. They blamed the activists

On average, an American uses more than 730 pounds of paper each year. About half of the wood used goes into paper products, such as boxes, stationery, computer printouts, napkins, and magazines. Some of these items contain recycled fiber, but most are still made from newly cut trees. Despite recycling efforts, paper still makes up about 40% of America's garbage.

Source: WoodWise (a program of Co-op America)

Read the Label

Worldwide, manufacturers make as much cloth from wood pulp as they do from wool. Rayon is the most common wood-based fabric, but acetate, triacetate, and Tencel® are also made from trees. Lots of water and chemicals are needed to extract usable fibers from trees; only about a third of the pulp obtained from a tree will end up in finished rayon thread. The resulting fabrics usually require dry cleaning, an added environmental concern. Much of the rayon purchased by Americans comes from developing countries, such as Indonesia, where environmental and labor laws are weak and poorly enforced.

Source: WoodWise

for the shutdown because they forced the government to restrict logging in the few areas of old-growth forest that are left. But that's not the real problem. The truth is the huge logging corporations have done so much clear-cutting in the last twenty years that they're running out of mature trees to cut down. The forest industry has become so focused on generating fast money for shareholders that it can't sustain itself anymore.

It wasn't always that way though. Up until the 1970s and '80s, most logging companies were small, family-run businesses. They worked the same areas for decades, selecting only mature trees for cutting and maintaining as much of the existing ecosystem as possible. It was a sustainable approach to forestry that provided steady jobs for local loggers and mills and didn't scar the landscape. But things started to change when big paper and lumber companies like Weyerhaeuser, Pacific Lumber, and Georgia Pacific started to buy up the small logging companies and their land holdings. All they saw was a huge untapped resource, hundreds of years in the making. They brought in new technologies to speed up the process, like mechanical tree-cutters that could cut down a tree and strip the branches in a fraction of the time it would take a couple of loggers with chainsaws. They cut new roads into the wilderness that allowed them to get at untouched forest areas. And they started clear-cutting. Pretty soon they had quadrupled the cut-rate and grabbed huge windfall profits for their shareholders. But it couldn't go on forever. Now we're down to just three to four per cent of the true old-growth forest we used to have, and we wouldn't even have that if it wasn't for the activists getting in the way.

Make no mistake, even with their acres of tree factories, the big paper and lumber corporations still have their eyes on the old-growth that's left. It's like gold to them, just sitting there; they'd love nothing more than to clear-cut all of it and make a pile of money in the process. In fact, areas of old-growth forest in the United States are probably more valuable today than any real estate in Beverly Hills. And don't expect our politicians to stand in their way, not when you've got lumber company executives with photos on their wall signed by Ronald Reagan, congratulating them for doing so much

for the U.S. economy. Big Timber spends just as much to keep Washington in line as the agri-corps, the chemical companies, and the oil companies.

I actually saw a photo just like that in Charles Hurwitz's living room. Charles Hurwitz was the CEO of a company called Maxxam at the time, and Maxxam was the principal shareholder in Pacific Lumber right around the time I was climbing the Golden Gate Bridge with my activist friends to protest the logging of ancient redwood trees in California. The banner we unfurled on top of the bridge actually read: "Hurwitz: Aren't Ancient Redwoods Worth More Than Gold?" We put that on the banner because Hurwitz was apparently fond of referring to the "Golden Rule" of business: "He who has the gold makes the rules."

Shortly after that demo, in 1997, Julia Butterfly Hill climbed up an ancient 200-foot-tall redwood tree on land owned by the Pacific Lumber Company near Stafford, California. She set up a little camp there for herself and determined to remain there until the company agreed not to cut down the trees. She would end up staying there for almost two years. A year in to her protest, because I was active in trying to save the old-growth forests, some of Julia's friends approached me to see if there was any way I could maybe intercede with Pacific Lumber and try to find a way for her to come down without anybody losing face. So I called up the head office to see if I could meet with Charles Hurwitz to discuss the problem.

Amazingly enough, we did arrange a meeting, and I jumped on a plane to Houston, where he lived, and went to see him at his penthouse apartment. The place was about what you would expect from a guy who ran a billion-dollar conglomerate: luxurious and beautifully decorated, but understated, not over-the-top like Donald Trump's place. Hurwitz met me at the door with his wife; we shook hands and went into the massive living room. The room had huge picture windows that were hermetically sealed from the outside like an office building, and they overlooked a beautiful park full of big, green, leafy trees, which I thought was rather fitting.

I sat down and he got me a drink and we made small talk while the chef prepared dinner. They asked me about my family and about show business and they told me about their family; it was all very pleasant, I must say. They had had their chef prepare a total vegan meal just for me, and we sat down and shared a wonderful dinner together. After dinner, Hurwitz led me off into the study where we had a couple more drinks and then, finally, we got around to discussing the situation with Julia and the redwoods.

We sat and talked for about an hour, just like two neighbors chatting over the fence, and by the time we were done, I liked him. I was embarrassed to admit it to any of my forest activist friends afterwards, but I friggin' liked the man. Before, when I was unfurling that banner on top of the Golden Gate, I was convinced that Hurwitz was the Antichrist, and you've pretty much got to believe that if you're going to go to so much trouble to single a guy out. But after I sat and talked to the man, I could see that he was a real guy. I could see that he had feelings and he cared about his family. He cared about making money too, obviously, and that's what he is certainly the best at, but I could see that money wasn't the only thing he cared about.

But as we began to get into it about harvesting the old-growth forests, I began to realize why it is that a basically good person can condone something so

wrong. He honestly did not grasp what his company was really doing to the environment. He knew they were cutting down a lot of trees, but he couldn't wrap his head around the kind of devastation that causes. In fact, I'm sure his nose is buried so far in his accounting books most of the time that he never looks out the window of his private plane to see the impact that clear-cutting has on the landscape.

He told me over and over again, and believed it, that "for every tree we cut down, we plant three others." So in his mind, he was actually increasing the tree population. I kept trying to explain to him that there is a difference between the trees his company plants and the ancient trees, but he just didn't get it.

At one point, he even said to me, "You know, if you don't cut down the big trees, the little trees underneath never get any sunlight so they never get a chance to grow."

I could not believe that one. I just shook my head and said, "Well, it's a good thing we're here to look after the little trees; I don't know how they got along for all those years without us."

For the most part, we agreed to disagree, and we left each other on relatively good terms I thought. We made some progress on the subject of Julia and I made the point I wanted to make, which was to ask him to make

Magazines

Approximately 12 billion magazines are printed annually in the U.S., consuming at least 2.2 million tons of paper each year, which requires more than 35 million trees. Less than 5% of magazine paper has any post-consumer recycled content.

Using factors such as the weight and the grade of paper used, size, number of pages, circulation, and frequency of publication, the Magazine Paper Project calculated the number of trees used by different magazines each year. Some examples:

People – 546,134 trees a year
Cosmopolitan – 328,577 trees a year
National Geographic – 505,819 trees a year

Source: Magazine Paper Project (a Co-op America program), August 29, 2002.

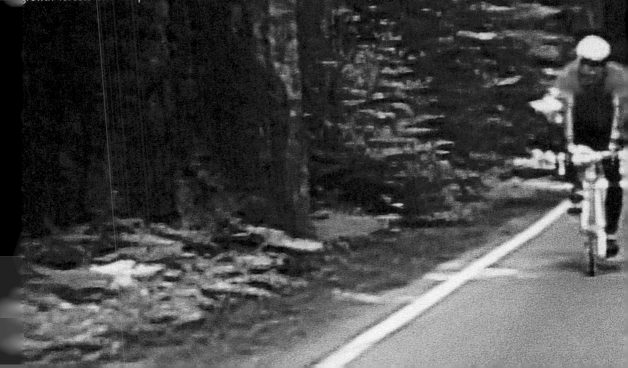

some effort at least to save the old-growth. He said he would try, but I honestly believe Hurwitz did not comprehend the severe consequences of his actions and the actions of his company. He couldn't make the "cause and effect" connection you have to make before you can lighten your footprint.

Right now, the only thing standing between old-growth forests and the logging companies are the people with enough guts to stand up and do something about it. It's extraordinary people like Julia Butterfly Hill, who ended up spending 738 days (1997–1999) living in the branches of that redwood tree so they couldn't chop it down. Maybe we all can't make that kind of commitment to the planet, but we can all do something. For starters, we can stop buying saunas, hot tubs, and patio furniture made from rare woods like redwood and teak when we know that's not good for the planet. Better yet, we can start using non-wood paper substitutes to blow our nose. Because the bottom line is this: we're either going to find an alternative source for paper and stop cutting down trees, or we're going to cut down all the trees and then find an alternative source for paper.

The good news is that we can get off the unsustainable path we're on and save what's left of our old-growth forests and unspoiled wilderness for our chil-dren. The first step is for each one of us to recognize the ways we encourage Big Timber to do what it does and cut back on our wood and paper product use. Paper tissues—not sustainable, use a handkerchief. Paper napkins—not sustainable, use a cloth napkin. Paper cups—not sustainable, use your own ceramic cup. You'll also find there are lots of recycled wood and paper products on the market now if you look for them.

If we can cut back on our demand for wood and paper, it might force the big logging companies to go back to the slower, more sustainable approach to tree harvesting that existed before the stock markets got involved. In fact, if we can force them to stop using mechanized tree cutters and bulldozers to wipe out whole forests, that might even create more jobs for traditional loggers; when you manage a forest sustainably, it actually takes more skill to go in and select trees for thinning and to avoid damaging the ecosystem. So I believe there's no reason why you can't still have jobs and a viable forest industry when you take a sustainable approach; hell, you can even buy "sustainably harvested" lumber at the Home Depot now. What you can't have, and what we can't afford any longer, are the massive spiked profits the big lumber companies reap from clear-cutting.

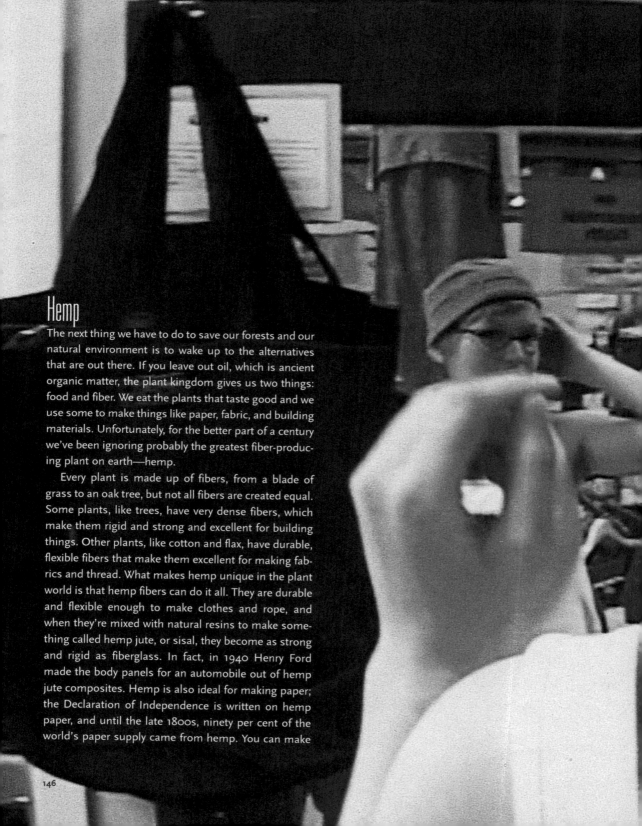

Hemp

The next thing we have to do to save our forests and our natural environment is to wake up to the alternatives that are out there. If you leave out oil, which is ancient organic matter, the plant kingdom gives us two things: food and fiber. We eat the plants that taste good and we use some to make things like paper, fabric, and building materials. Unfortunately, for the better part of a century we've been ignoring probably the greatest fiber-producing plant on earth—hemp.

Every plant is made up of fibers, from a blade of grass to an oak tree, but not all fibers are created equal. Some plants, like trees, have very dense fibers, which make them rigid and strong and excellent for building things. Other plants, like cotton and flax, have durable, flexible fibers that make them excellent for making fabrics and thread. What makes hemp unique in the plant world is that hemp fibers can do it all. They are durable and flexible enough to make clothes and rope, and when they're mixed with natural resins to make something called hemp jute, or sisal, they become as strong and rigid as fiberglass. In fact, in 1940 Henry Ford made the body panels for an automobile out of hemp jute composites. Hemp is also ideal for making paper; the Declaration of Independence is written on hemp paper, and until the late 1800s, ninety per cent of the world's paper supply came from hemp. You can make

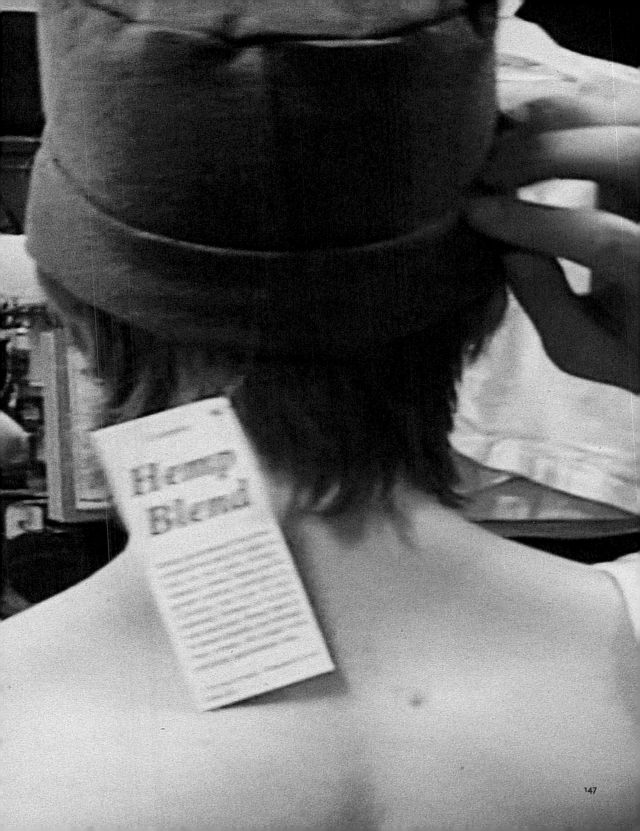

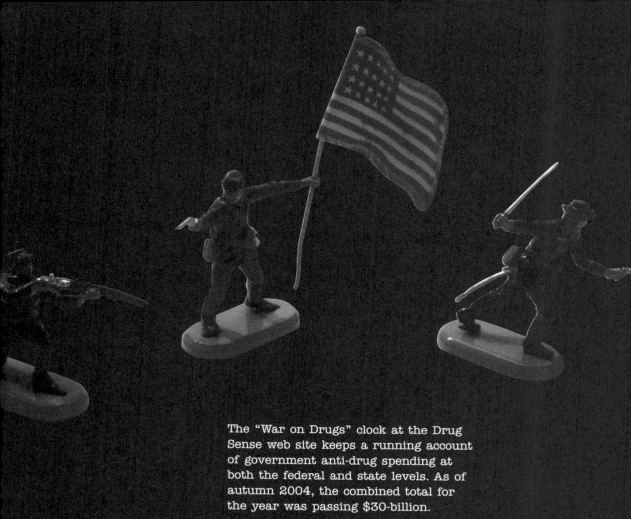

The "War on Drugs" clock at the Drug Sense web site keeps a running account of government anti-drug spending at both the federal and state levels. As of autumn 2004, the combined total for the year was passing $30-billion.

Source: Drug Sense

medicines with it, as well as plastic, cosmetics, paint. Shit, on the SOL Tour we drove a coach bus from Seattle to Long Beach burning nothing but hemp seed oil. If that's not a miracle plant, I'd like to know what is.

In fact, just about the only thing you can't do with industrial hemp is get high off it. Although it does come from exactly the same plant family as Mary-J, it only produces very low levels of tetrahydrocannabinol, better known as THC, which is the psychoactive ingredient in pot that makes college students laugh uncontrollably and want to eat bags of Cheetos when they smoke it. Industrial hemp doesn't do that; if it did, the Pilgrims probably would've smoked all the ropes on the Mayflower long before they landed at Plymouth Rock.

So the next question is, why isn't the human race, especially in the developed world, taking advantage of probably the most sustainable source of fiber on the planet? A better question might be, who bene-

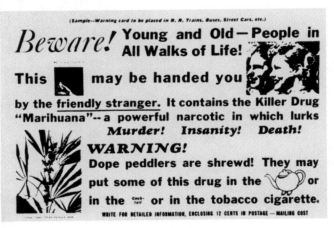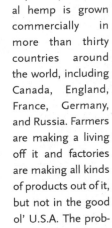

(Sample--Warning card to be placed in R. R. Trains, Buses, Street Cars, etc.)

Beware! Young and Old—People in All Walks of Life!

This ■ may be handed you by the <u>friendly stranger.</u> It contains the Killer Drug "Marihuana"-- a powerful narcotic in which lurks Murder! Insanity! Death!

WARNING!
Dope peddlers are shrewd! They may put some of this drug in the 🫖 or in the ▦ or in the tobacco cigarette.

WRITE FOR DETAILED INFORMATION, ENCLOSING 12 CENTS IN POSTAGE — MAILING COST

fits from our *not* using it? Well, if you remove a primary fiber crop from our farms, you put artificial pressure on our forests to provide fiber for paper and wood fiber products like particleboard and paneling, and that helps the timber industry. If you rely on cotton and synthetic fibers to make thread and fabric, the chemical companies benefit, both because they manufacture the synthetics and because today half of all agricultural pesticides are used in cotton production. If you convince Henry Ford to use sheet metal panels to make car bodies instead of cheaper hemp jute, that helps the steel industry. And if you discourage the use of alternative fuels made from hemp and other plants—well, we all know who benefits there.

We've been doing all these things for a hundred years now while a useful, totally renewable resource like industrial hemp sat on the shelf. How many more acres of old-growth forest would we have today if we had been using hemp to make paper for the last hundred years? How much less air pollution would we have today if the auto industry had been committed to developing engine technology using fuels made from hemp, corn, or even methane gas from pig shit? There was always a better way, we just allowed powerful interests to lead us down the wrong path.

But that's OK; now that we see the error of our ways our society can start taking advantage of a miracle plant like hemp, right? Wrong. Not in the United States, anyway. Today, industrial hemp is grown commercially in more than thirty countries around the world, including Canada, England, France, Germany, and Russia. Farmers are making a living off it and factories are making all kinds of products out of it, but not in the good ol' U.S.A. The problem, of course, is that industrial hemp is just too closely related to the cannabis plant, which has been known to produce a feeling of euphoria if smoked or ingested, and the U.S. government has a real problem with people being euphoric. In fact, the government has invested billions and billions of dollars and millions of hours of effort over the last seventy years to do their damnedest to make sure nobody got happy smoking that "Mexican Killer Weed."

Hemp has been grown in the United States since long before the pilgrims got here, and they grew a shitload of it themselves. George Washington even grew hemp at Mount Vernon. All the bullshit surrounding hemp didn't start until 1933; that's when the U.S. government finally admitted that you can't stop people, especially white people, from doing something they really want to do and

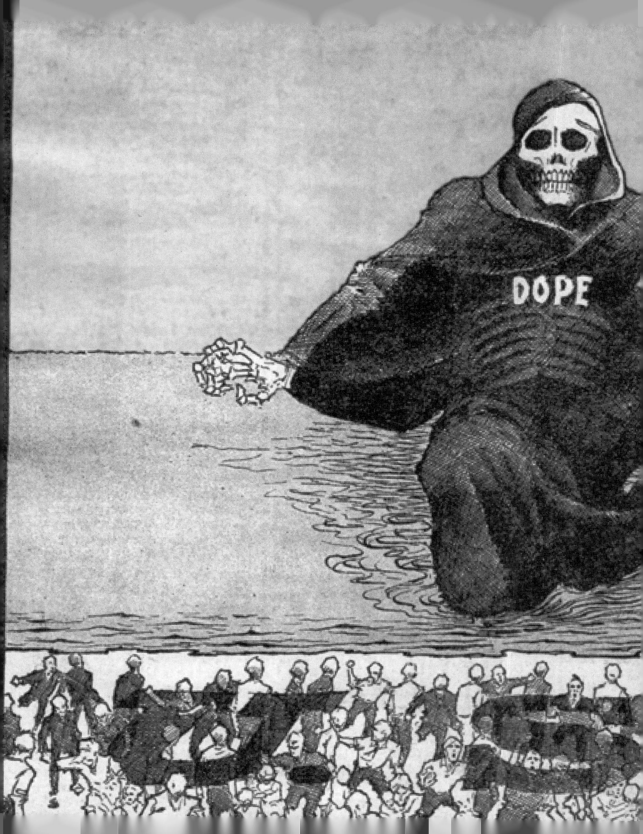

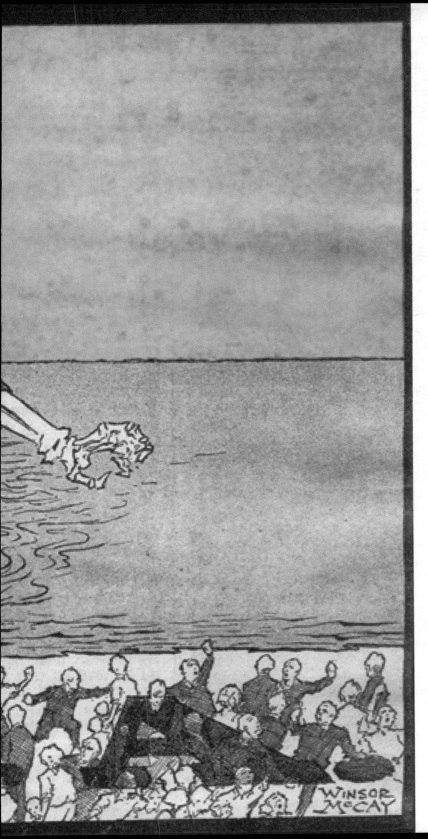

repealed the Prohibition Act. The problem was they had all these federal lawmen on their hands who had nothing to do now that the bootleggers were legit. So they transferred them over to the Federal Bureau of Narcotics (which was created in 1930 and later morphed into the DEA) and put them to work chasing down Native Americans, black jazz musicians, and Mexican migrant workers for smoking "reefer."

The joke is, up until that point, marijuana was never a problem in the U.S. Very few people even knew what it was, and doctors regularly prescribed it to patients with nervous disorders. But the Feds needed to justify their law enforcement budgets and reefer was it. Using propaganda films like *Reefer Madness,* they tried to spread fear about "the demon weed." They said reefer could twist people's minds so much that they could commit murder. They said it would cause young people to riot. It could even make a white woman so wild with lust, they said, that she might forget herself and climb into bed with a black man. Unfortunately, they didn't bother to make any distinction between the stuff you smoke and the stuff you can make shit out of.

In 1937, they passed the Marihuana Tax Act, which on the face of it seemed to impose a small licensing fee on those who wanted to grow and sell marijuana, but through tricky clauses made it effectively impossible to grow or sell marijuana or its relative, hemp, legally. That only succeeded in pushing the production of the potent weed underground, but it completely wiped out the production of industrial hemp. It's probably just a coincidence that this happened right around the same time that the DuPont company was trying to introduce a revolutionary new "synthetic" fiber called nylon to the textile market.

So industrial hemp, with all its potential benefits, was put in mothballs in the 1930s and it's still there today. It did make a small comeback during World War II, when the Feds realized they were running out of rope for the war effort. They were so desperate that in 1942 they even made a propaganda film called *Hemp*

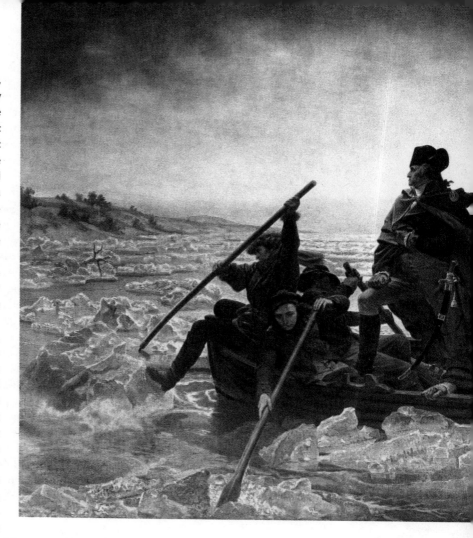

For Victory that encouraged farmers to plant hemp. The film talked about "the wonder plant" and all the products you can make from it. It even said it was patriotic to grow hemp, if you can believe that. As soon as the war was over though, hemp was Public Enemy Number One again.

As for the seventy-year-long fight against pot—well, we all know how that's going. President after president has tried to wipe it out, but I guess there are just too many black jazz musicians around to keep the demand up. Nixon tried to seal off the Mexican border in the 60s; Ford tried to poison the evil pot smokers with paraquat in the 70s; Reagan declared war on it in the 80s; and George Bush, Sr., spent something like $12-billion fighting it into the 90s. And petit Bush, the Shrub

Monkey? Maybe the reason he's not so vocal about is he probably smoked a fair amount of the shit himself before he found Jesus.

Well guess what? The fight to save us all from "reefer madness" has been a big sham. Seventy years later, we've still got pot. We've always had pot. What we haven't had are the benefits of industrial hemp. Meanwhile, it turns out we didn't need all our paper to come from trees, we didn't need all our fuel to come from petroleum, and we didn't need thread and fabric to come from chemical synthetics and pesticide-laden cotton. What an incredible waste of time.

The opponents of hemp always argue that encouraging hemp production is a slippery slope toward the

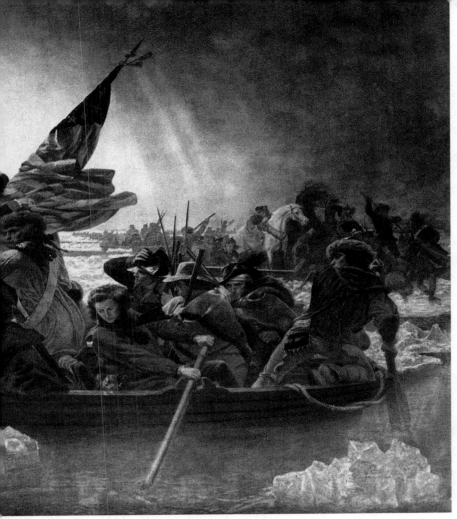

Disease Control and Prevention) or get killed through drunk driving (17,000 in 2003 according to the NHTSA). Heart disease and cancer are two of the biggest killers in the world today, and we know cigarette smoking is the main cause of both, yet cigarettes are legal. Alcoholism leads to all kinds of social problems, yet alcohol is legal. Thousands more people die each year because they become addicted to prescription drugs, yet prescription drugs are legal. Marijuana is not addictive and, as far as I know, it has never killed anybody (many a night I've tried to O.D.), but our jails are full of people who dare to use that non-corporate drug.

What all this bullshit has to do with an innocuous weed like industrial hemp I'll never know. But when you cut away the crap, hemp is just one example of the sustainable alternative resources we've managed to ignore for decades now. There are lots of others, things like wind power and solar power have always been right there, waiting for us to take full advantage of them, but again and again we let the Beast distract us and pull us off course.

We can't afford to be distracted any longer, because right now we're on course for an ecological meltdown on this planet. The developed nations of the world—the "First World," which includes North America, Europe, Australia, New Zealand, and a few countries in Asia—currently have about twenty per cent of the earth's pop-

legalization of marijuana, as if people would hide their herb in a hemp patch after telling the government where it is. But I see them as two separate issues. Whether or not you believe in the legalization of marijuana (personally, I think in a free country you should be allowed to do what you want as long as you don't harm anyone else), I don't think that has anything to do with exploring sustainable alternatives, although both sides try to use the pot issue to cloud the argument.

They even try to make smoking pot a health issue, but if the government was really concerned about people's health, you'd think they'd try to do something about all the people who die from smoking cigarettes (400,000 Americans a year, according to the Centers for

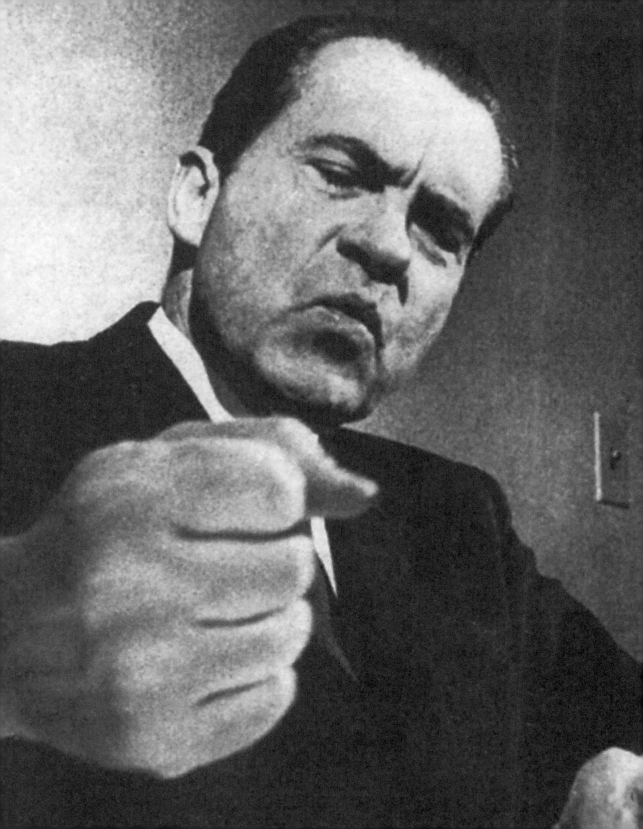

ulation but use up about eighty per cent of the resources and create more than fifty per cent of the pollution. The countries with the biggest populations, meanwhile, the "Third World" countries, put relatively little strain on the planet. But that's changing fast.

Two countries that we in the West have always thought of as Third World or developing countries, India and China, account for almost a sixth of the world's population between them, and their economies are growing. People in those countries see American movies and TV shows, and they want to live like people live in the developed world, and who can blame them? The problem is, look at the damage to our planet being caused by just twenty per cent of the human population living our unsustainable Western lifestyle. Imagine if, fifty or seventy-five years from now, half of the world's population is living that lifestyle—millions more people burning fossil fuels; millions more using petroleum-based products; millions more using wood and paper products; millions more using products made with synthetic chemicals; and millions of new factories and industries pumping poison into the air, the water, and ground in places with little or no regulation. And who the hell are we to tell them not to do it? After all, we've been doing it in the West for years. Also, many (if not most) of those pollution-belching factories are owned by western interests.

Obviously it's going to be over for this planet if we let it come to that. And most of us may not give a shit today because we'll all be dead in fifty years, but our kids would probably appreciate it if we changed course now, and our grandkids would for sure.

There were times on the SOL Tour, usually when I was riding past a big clear-cut, when I could feel my spirit sinking pretty low. It's a sight that really stays with you, haunting you, and it's just that much worse when you're aware of the fact that it's all so unnecessary. I'd always get a lift, though, when I'd get past the carnage and back among the trees, and not just because trees make a better windbreak than a clear-cut. You could just feel the presence of these powerful, ancient beings around you. Sometimes, when I was chugging uphill on a steep grade, I used to imagine the trees pumping out oxygen for me, lending me their energy and helping me up the hill. I believe we can all get energy from nature if we open ourselves up to it, in the same way we get energy from our family and friends. That's what keeps me going.

I remember riding through this one beautiful grove of trees one particular morning. There was a dense fog, like a cloud had settled down right among the trees, and beams of sunlight were streaming through all around, making patches of light here and there on the ground. It was so beautiful and peaceful. Then I noticed a sign just off the road; it said this was a "private forest," owned by a major paper company. I couldn't help but think that that magical grove of trees was destined to become wood pulp one day, and I'm not ashamed to say I had tears in my eyes when I rode off.

Another time I was riding through another beautiful grove of trees when I saw another little sign off by the side of the road. This one said "Edith Reinhart Grove." The sign went on to say how she was one of a number of people who had contributed money so that this small piece of forest could be bought up and preserved in its natural state forever. Now I don't know who Edith Reinhart is—in fact, she's probably gone by now and I'll never get to meet her—but as I stood there under those tall trees, the sunlight shimmering on the forest floor, I thought to myself, "Man, if all she ever did was save these trees, old Edith really did something pretty magnificent with her life."

A little later that same day we came out of the forest and turned onto a big highway that was clogged with logging trucks. They had cleared the trees back for about a hundred yards on either side of the highway. The ditches were full of trash and, every so often, a dead deer or elk killed by a logging truck. There was a big sign at the side of the road that read, "William G. Heighe Memorial Highway"; I guess he was some politician years ago who made sure that that highway got built to encourage industry in the area.

As I peddled off down the road, I remember I turned to my brother and said, "If you're still around after I die and for some reason somebody decides they want to name something after me, do me a favor and please make sure it's a grove of trees and not a highway."

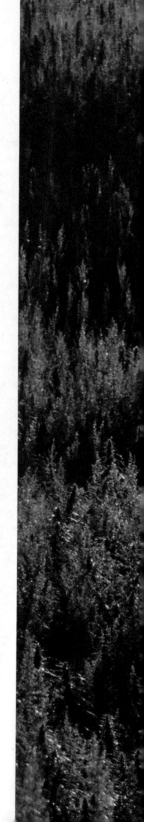

HIGH TIME FOR HEMP

Paul Armentano

"The marketplace, not myopic rules, should determine hemp's future in America."
—*New York Times* Editorial Board, April 11, 1998

Imagine a cash crop that farmers could grow every hundred days without using pesticides, and that manufacturers could employ in more than 25,000 environmentally friendly products. Now imagine that the federal government was spending millions of dollars every year to eradicate this plant and criminally prosecute those who grow it. Sadly, we don't have to imagine such a scenario. The plant is hemp, and for the tens of thousands of American farmers who could benefit from its legal cultivation, the Feds' prejudicial policy regarding its industrial use is all too real.

What is Hemp?

Hemp is a distinct variety of the plant species *Cannabis sativa* that contains minimal amounts (less than one per cent) of tetrahydrocannabinol (THC), the primary psychoactive ingredient in marijuana. Often referred to as pot's "misunderstood cousin," hemp is a tall, slender, fibrous plant similar to flax or kenaf. Farmers around the globe have cultivated hemp for fiber and food for nearly 12,000 years, and American colonialists relied on the crop as a raw material for making paper, oil, and rope. Today, various parts of the plant can be used in the manufacturing of textiles, paper, paint, clothing, plastics, cosmetics, foodstuffs, insulation, animal feed, and countless other products.

For modern farmers, hemp remains a low-maintenance crop with big advantages. The plant is especially hardy (it's a weed, after all), may be grown in almost any climate, and produces a much higher yield-per-acre than more common linen substitutes like cotton. In addition, because hemp plants typically grow from six to sixteen feet tall, the resulting shade blocks out competing weeds, allowing farmers to reduce their use of herbicides. Lastly, hemp has an average growing cycle of only one hundred days and leaves the soil virtually weed-free for the next planting.

Hemp in the twenty-first century is harvested for commercial purposes in over thirty nations, including Australia, China, Japan, Canada, and countries in the European Union. The Canadian government issued about 240 hemp production licenses in 2002 alone. In the United States, however, hemp remains Public Enemy Number One.

Although the hemp plant still grows wild across much of America and presents no public health or safety threat (smoking it won't give you a buzz but it may give you a headache), police departments nevertheless spend millions of dollars and thousands of man-hours every year eradicating it. According to Drug Enforcement Administration (DEA) records, ninety-eight percent of all the marijuana eliminated annually by law enforcement is actually hemp. That's right; rather than tapping the extraordinary potential of this self-sustaining agricultural resource, the Feds are spending your hard-earned tax dollars to destroy it.

erica's Hempen History

asn't always like this. There once was a time when erica's political leaders—men such as George hington and Thomas Jefferson—espoused the es of hemp, calling its production necessary for the lth and protection of the country." Several towns and es—such as Hempstead, New York, and Hemphill, —were even named after the lucrative crop.

August 1937, however, everything changed.

Congress had re...serted its total ban on her tion. That federal ban remains in effect today

Nevertheless, a domestic hemp industry continues to grow in America despite the gov bureaucratic moratorium. Today, U.S. reta manufacturers annually import approximate. lion pounds of hemp fiber, 450,000 pounds seeds, and 331 pounds of hempseed oil fror and other nations that regulate hemp farming law permits the importation of hempen prod

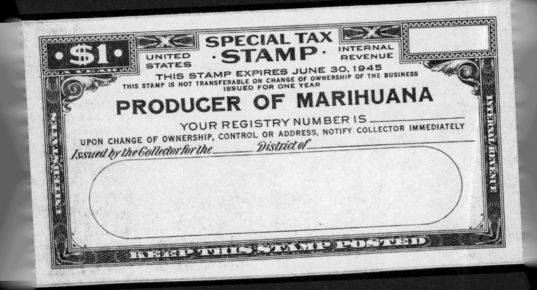

g just one hour of legislative debate, Congress e Marihuana Tax Act, which tolled the death he once prominent industry.

looked bleak for hemp farmers, that is until r II. After Japanese military conquests in Asia of the world's rope-fiber supply in enemy e U.S. government once again turned to emp production to come to our nation's res sands of farmers grew fields of federally sub emp to fulfill America's wartime needs. ely, when World War II ended, so did the gov tolerance of hemp cultivation. By 1957

fiber, and sterilized seeds.) In addition, a growing ber of health professionals are praising the nutri value of hemp, noting that hemp seeds are secono to soy in protein and contain the highest concentr of essential amino and fatty acids of any food.

Given such a strong and diverse résumé, it's no der hemp has been endorsed by the likes of the Agriculture Department's Alternative Agricult Research and Commercialization Center, the Natic Conference of State Legislatures, environmental acti and Green Party presidential candidate Ralph Na and health guru Andrew Weil.

Where Does the U.S. Government Stand on Hemp?

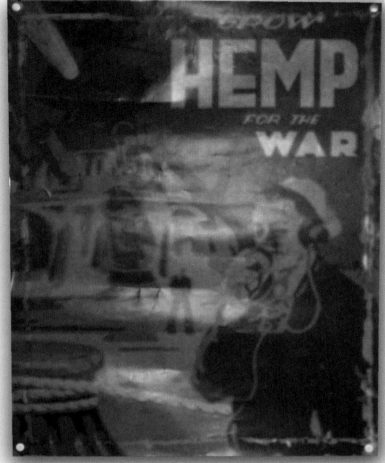

In a word: opposed. Despite hemp's emergence as a worldwide industry, the DEA and the White House Office of National Drug Control Policy (a.k.a. the Drug Czar's office) remain unwilling to even debate the issue. Currently, only the DEA has the power to license farmers to legally grow hemp, even in those states where local laws permit it. But, predictably, they have denied virtually every permit for large-scale hemp farming within America's borders for the last four decades. (The lone exception to this rule came in 1999, when the DEA granted Hawaii researchers permission to grow a one-quarter-acre test plot of the crop.)

In a 1995 USDA White Paper, the DEA stated that they are "opposed to any consideration of hemp as a legitimate fiber or pulp product." Since then, White House and DEA officials have stonewalled several state efforts to enact hemp cultivation and research bills by threatening to arrest farmers who attempt to grow it—even in cases where such cultivation is in compliance with state laws. Even more disturbing, in 1999 DEA officials ordered U.S. Customs officials to begin illegally seizing sterilized hemp seeds as they entered the country. The agency later backed down after threats from the Canadian embassy and commercial seed producers.

More recently, DEA officials attempted to sabotage the blossoming hemp foods industry by issuing a ban on all hemp food and oil products containing even trace amounts of THC. The DEA issued the ban despite a Department of Justice finding that such products are specifically excluded from regulation under the Controlled Substances Act. In response to the DEA's

action, lawyers for the Hemp Industries Association (HIA) and seven hemp food companies filed suit against the agency with the Ninth Circuit Court of Appeals in San Francisco urging the court to enjoin the regulations. In addition, a Canadian hemp manufacturer, Kenex Limited, filed suit with the U.S. State Department arguing that the ban violates provisions of the North American Free Trade Agreement (NAFTA) and illegally undermines its ability to do business. Kenex is seeking $20-million from the U.S. government in compensatory damages. HIA won its suit against the DEA in February 2004; the Kenex suit is pending at this writing but both it and the HIA ruling will have ramifications for future U.S. hemp policy.

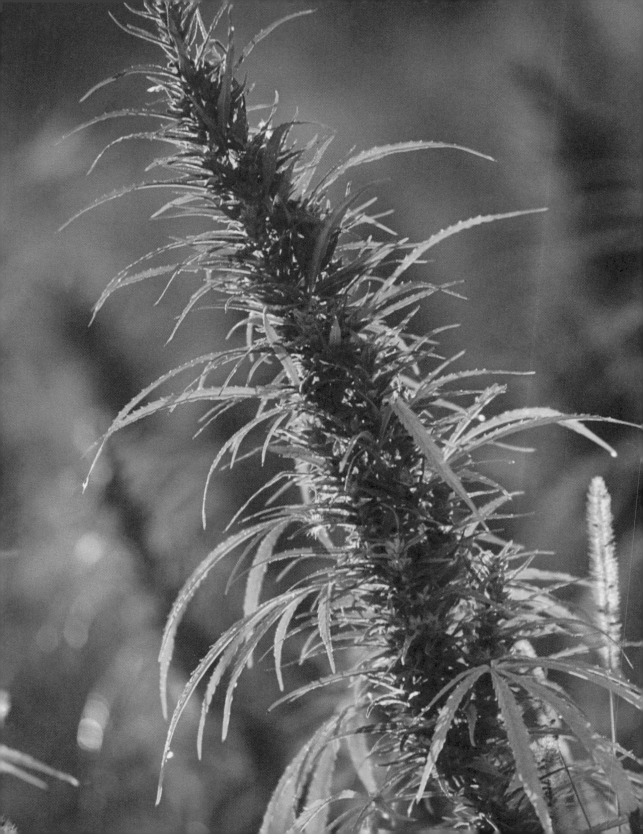

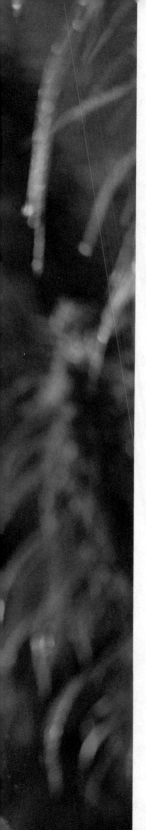

Hemp Today

Although the federal government refuses to waver in its enforcement of hemp prohibition, public, state, and international support for legalization continues to grow. The European Union currently subsidizes farmers to grow hemp, and the plant is now legally recognized as a commercial crop in many of the world's prominent economic treaties, including the North American Free Trade Agreement (NAFTA) and the General Agreement on Tariffs and Trade (GATT).

In recent years, a number of U.S. states have commissioned studies recommending hemp as a viable economic crop. A 1995 study by the University of Kentucky estimated that local farmers could earn roughly $320 per acre growing hemp for straw and grain, and $340 an acre from growing certified hemp seed. Similar state-sponsored studies in Illinois and North Dakota concluded that hemp's profit potential warranted immediately amending state and federal law. Accordingly, three states—North Dakota, Montana, and West Virginia—have passed legislation legalizing hemp cultivation by licensed farmers. Several others have passed resolutions demanding Congress rescind their archaic and myopic ban on hemp. And for once, it appears as if Washington may be listening.

For the first time ever, there is a push in Congress to remove hemp regulation from the authority of the DEA and place it in the hands of the U.S. Department of Agriculture. In addition, several representatives in Congress are also speaking out against the DEA's efforts to ban hemp foods and seeds. A "Dear Colleague" letter by Reps. George Miller of California and Ron Paul of Texas noted that, "The DEA should encourage the development and use of [hemp] products and not set unwarranted barriers to their production." The letter further urged Congress and the DEA to "follow the lead of other countries" which have enacted legal distinctions between hemp and non-industrial varieties of cannabis.

Unfortunately, there still remains far too much ignorance regarding the economic and agricultural advantages of industrial hemp. And that is where you come in. America's hemp revival is a "grassroots" movement (pardon the pun) spearheaded by people just like you who care about economic justice and environmental sustainability. They are people like you who write letters to their local paper, lobby their politicians and farm bureaus, and support their local hemp businesses. They are people like you who make, and have made, a difference in the way our nation views its most misunderstood crop. And they are people like you, who will ultimately pave the way for the return of one of America's most time-tested and versatile agricultural resources.

Paul Armentano is a senior policy analyst for NORML and The NORML Foundation (www.norml.org) in Washington, DC. His work has previously appeared in the following anthologies: Busted: Stone Cowboys, Narco-Lords and Washington's War on Drugs (Nations Books, 2002); You Are Being Lied To: The Disinformation Guide to Media Distortion, Historical Whitewashes and Cultural Myths (Disinformation Books, 2001); and Drug Abuse: Opposing Viewpoints (Greenhaven Press, 1999). He has previously testified on the hemp issue before the U.S. Department of Agriculture and the U.S. Department of Justice.

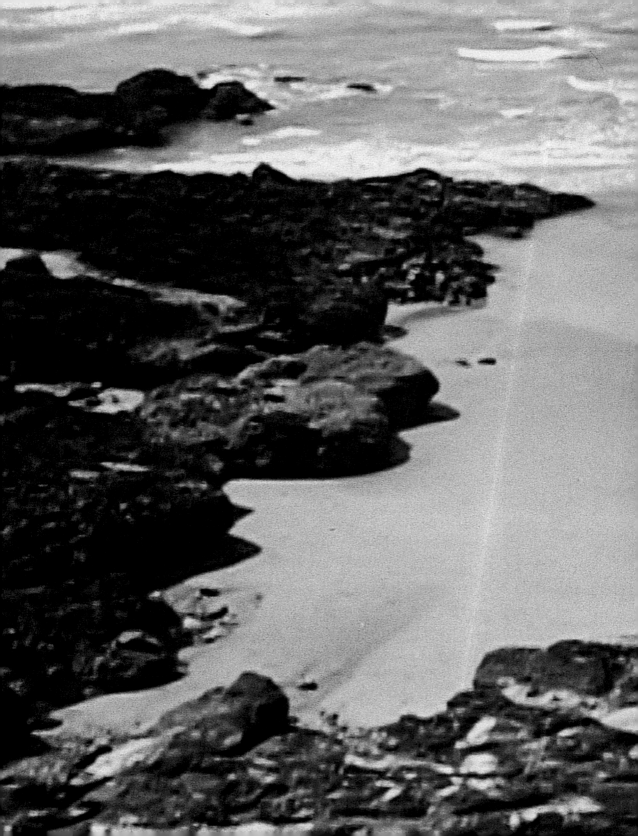

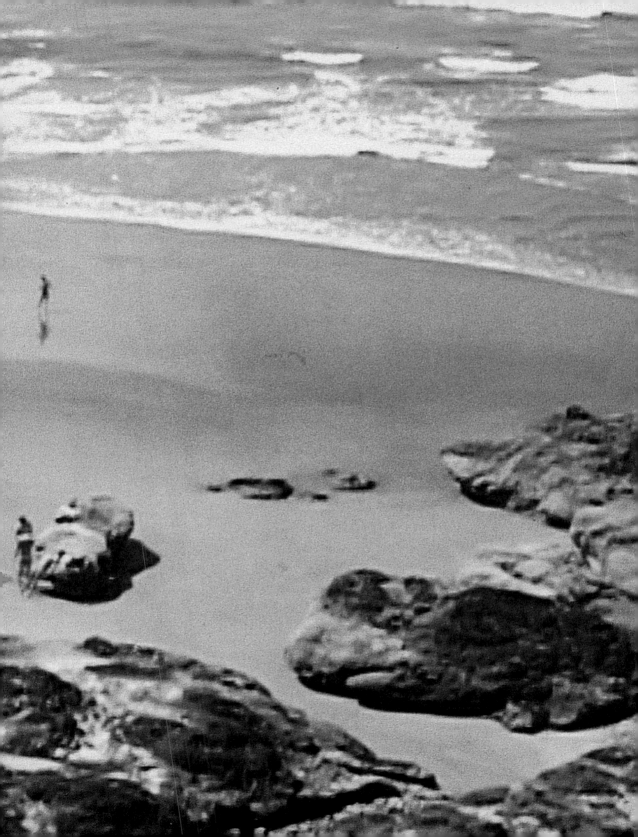

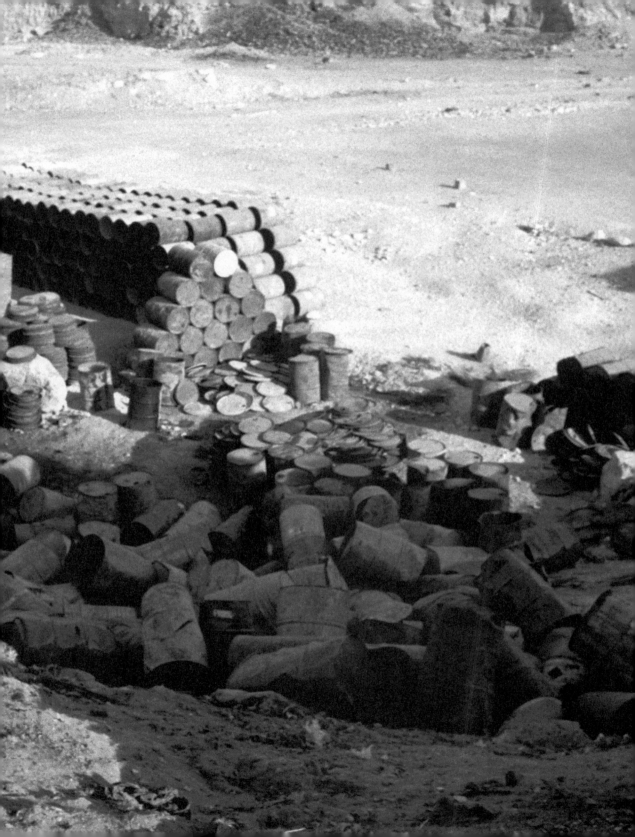

CONNECTING

I believe all people, at least once in their life, should take the time to go on a really long bike trip or a long hike. You could just pick a highway, like we did on the SOL Tour, and ride as far as you can for a week or so, or you could hike the Appalachian Trail or something like it for a few days. Believe me, you learn a few things about the planet when you travel over it slowly that you tend to miss when you're speeding along in a car or flying over at 30,000 feet.

The first thing that hits you is how incredibly beautiful our planet is—the birds, the trees, the mountains, the ocean. It's like their natural beauty is amplified when you're just out there being a small part of it, not hidden behind a layer of something man-made. Unfortunately, you also see a lot of bad stuff too. You can see signs of the negative impact of modern human activity on the planet almost everywhere. On our bike trip, I saw up close the damage done by things like clear -cutting, strip-mining, factory farming, and hydroelectric dams. It was a real wake-up call for me, and I've been wide awake ever since.

If I came away from that experience with anything, it's the knowledge that the capacity for our planet to sustain life is under attack. When I tell people about my experience, a lot of them say that it's a deliberate attack by the multi-national corporations and I agree, that's definitely part of it. Other people say that it's the result of the greed of western society, and I think that that's definitely part of it too—God knows, there's lots of blame to go around. But the bottom line is, if God made us stewards of the earth, she's pissed. It's time to stop looking for someone to blame and start doing something about it. That means each one of us, individually.

When you think about it, humans have only been doing the fossil fuel thing for a few hundred years, and only in a really serious way for about the last hundred. That's a split-second when you think about how long this planet has existed. But look how much damage we've managed to cause in just that miniscule amount of time. The scientific community has been trying to tell us for years that the negative fallout from our dependence on fossil fuels is starting to show up everywhere. From the Himalayan glaciers to the Antarctic, the planet is calling for help. And I think when DDT starts showing up in the polar ice cap (which also happens to be melting from the greenhouse effect), it's time to start listening. It's like we're determined to punch holes in the bottom of the boat we're all sailing in.

Probably the most obvious sign that burning fossil fuels is killing the planet is global warming. We have satellite images that show chunks of the polar ice cap as big as some states breaking off and starting to melt. But people don't want to make the connection between that and their SUV. We experience record heat waves in Europe and North America and how do we respond? By cranking up the air conditioning and making it even worse. In fact, the heat has made us suck so hard on the system at times that we end up shutting the system down. And how do the Texas oil men respond when you suggest we might be heading in the wrong direction? They say we need more scientific study to determine if there really is a "greenhouse effect." I say all you need to do is walk outside; you don't need a scientist to tell you the temperature's rising.

Global warming is something we can all see, or at least something we *should* see. The planet is sending out all kinds of subtle signals to let us know that things just aren't right. For years, scientists have documented a worldwide decline in many frog and salamander species, which are a bellwether of ecological health. We lose millions of acres of old-growth forest every year to acid rain caused by air pollution from factories, and that's in addition to the acres of forest they chop down to make grazing land for beef cattle in places like Brazil and the thousands of trees that are destroyed just to print the *New York Times* every day. Coral reefs are retreating. Sea levels are rising. That's the sad state of the world today, and if you ask me, we don't need any more scientific studies to figure out if we're moving in the right direction.

Just think about water, the very essence of life on this planet. Up until well into the last century, you could still drink water straight from streams in wilderness areas of North America. I don't think there are too many people who would be quick to do that today, no matter where the stream was. And I don't know anybody who doesn't think twice about drinking water straight out of the tap anymore (ironically, some of the worse things in our water are put there by the government—chlorine and fluoride). That's the sad truth of it, and we should all be a little bothered by the fact we have to walk around today with little plastic bottles of drinkable water, especially since the same folks who polluted the water now make bucks every time we buy their bottled variety.

The fact is, there are very few places, if any, left in the world that haven't been touched in some way by fossil fuel consumption and pollution. I don't think it's possible to name one country, certainly not in the developed world, where industries don't pump pollutants into the air and water, where you can't find even trace amounts of dangerous chemicals in plants, marine life, and land animals. And those pollutants and chemicals are transmitted via plants and animals to humans. Today, courtesy of pollution and fossil fuels, we can find toxins in the food we eat, the water we drink, and the air we breathe. In the U.S., one of every two men and one in every three women will develop cancer in their lifetime. One out of every two people will develop heart disease. The World Health Organization (WHO) estimates that 600,000 people die from the effects of air pollution each year worldwide. You think maybe there's some kind of connection there? It's no wonder people like that show *Survivor* so much; we can all relate.

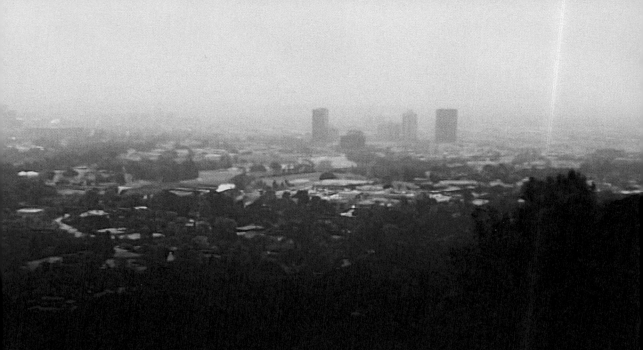

As I say, humans haven't really been sucking the fossil fuel teat for that long, so we can be forgiven, I guess, for maybe the first hundred and fifty years or so of stupidity. It took us at least that long to figure out that maybe total dependence on fossil fuels wasn't such a great idea after all. Since the middle of the last century, though, there's been no excuse. But we just pig-headedly continue to move down an unsustainable path that can only lead to our own destruction.

A perfect example of that kind of human stupidity is the city of Los Angeles, a place where I've spent quite a lot of time over the years. I read in a book one time that until World War II, Los Angeles was a nice, quiet, clean place on the ocean with a population of about half a million. After the war though, literally millions of people descended on the Los Angeles area looking for work and the whole California lifestyle, and ninety per cent of them brought a car. Obviously, all these people needed somewhere to live, so the L.A. area developed really quickly as this sprawling urban center with huge disconnected suburbs. And because the city didn't want the responsibility of moving all these new people around, lots of big roads and highways were built so people could get around in their cars. Public transit wasn't even an afterthought; the car companies paved

over mass transit in L.A. Well, anyone who has ever been to L.A. knows they're paying for those decisions today, in the form of smog and traffic gridlock. But L.A. is just one example; there are lots of other cities designed to suit industry and the automobile, rather than people.

So if we can't tear down places like L.A. and start from scratch, what can we do to make our planet more sustainable and more livable? Well, we can start by acknowledging that continuing to build our society around the consumption of fossil fuels is just insane. We can start to see the notion of cheap fossil fuel energy for what it is, a lie, because the environmental and health costs aren't factored in at the pump, not to mention the billions a year in subsidies and tax breaks. We can start to explore sustainable alternatives in our personal lives and support politicians who want to move our society in that direction. If we don't, our children and our grandchildren can expect to fight more wars in the Persian Gulf over increasingly limited resources while the air over L.A. turns blacker by the day.

I saw a commercial on television recently for one of the big oil companies that almost made me choke on my celery stick. It had this attractive woman in it who was supposed to be an environmental engineer working for the oil company and she was talking about everything the company was doing to protect wildlife and wilderness areas in Alaska where they were drilling. It just so happens that this was the same oil company that had a little accident with one of their tankers off the coast of Alaska a few years back and beaches in the area are still contiminated with oil. But she didn't mention that.

That kind of bullshit makes me crazy because that's how the Beast hypnotizes people into allowing it to keep doing what it's doing. The corporations say they care because they know people don't like to see sea birds covered in crude oil. And that makes it OK for you to drive your SUV as long as you know they're doing their best to keep the oil off the birds. But they don't care—not the oil companies, not the lumber companies, not the chemical companies, none of them. If we let them, they'll pollute every bit of it; they'll take every tree; they'll poison every stream. If we leave it up to big industry, every breath of air you take into your lungs will be toxic. The Beast is kidnapping our Mother Earth, and I think we need to crawl up into the belly of the Beast and give it a high colonic and a wheatgrass implant.

But make no mistake: the transition from an unsustainable lifestyle to a sustainable lifestyle is going to take some effort. In order to wean ourselves off the corporate teat, we're going to have to start to reestablish the connections that we've lost over the years, like the one between the food we eat and our health, and the one between human activity and the health of the planet.

The unsustainable approach only works if you break those connections and isolate everything in your mind. The logging industry, for example, argues that they plant more trees than they cut down, so clear-cutting old-growth forests doesn't matter. But that approach ignores the fact there are other plants and animals that live in those old-growth forests; it's a whole ecosystem where each part is dependent on the others for survival. If you cut down the old-growth, you can't replace it, but we've come to think in such isolated terms that we don't see the repercussive effects of each and every thing we do. We need to start making those connections again.

I remember riding by myself on the SOL Tour through an area of beautiful old-growth forest in Oregon when I came around a corner and found a big bag of garbage broken open in the middle of the road. I guess somebody was driving along in their Lincoln Navigator and decided it was time to clean the beer cans, coffee cups, and cigarette butts out of the front seat. So they filled up a plastic bag and just rolled down the window and dropped it. Obviously they didn't care what happened to the garbage after they chucked it out the window; their personal space was a little cleaner, and that was all that mattered to them.

I stopped and picked up the trash that was spread across the road and tried to put it back in what was left of the bag, then I carried it to the next rest stop along the highway and put it in a trash can. As I put the bag in the can, I thought to myself, "How fucking hard was that?" But some people just don't make the connection. The

Global Warming

- Since 1900, the mean surface temperature of the earth has increased by about 1.1°F (0.6°Celsius).
- Over the last 40 years (the period with the most reliable data) the temperature increased by about 0.5°F (0.2–0.3°Celsius).
- The Arctic ice pack has lost about 40% of its thickness over the past four decades.
- The global sea level rose about three times faster over the past 100 years than in the previous 3,000 years.
- A growing number of studies show that plants and animals are changing their range and behavior in response to climate change.

Source: Union of Concerned Scientists

ones who dumped that bag of garbage out of their car thought they were removing it from their environment, but they forgot that the whole planet is their environment. Not only that, they forgot it's my environment too, and yours. Making connections—that's what it's all about.

Another time, I was in New York visiting an actor friend of mine and he was showing me around his new loft in this classy refurbished warehouse in TriBeCa. He introduced me to the guy who owned the place, who gave me the tour and insisted that we go down to the basement to see this magnificent bar he was building. When we got down there, the guy was going around bragging about how much everything in the bar cost and how he went to Europe to buy this, and to Japan to buy that.

Eventually, he took me over to this beautiful wooden stage he had built and, jumping up on it, he says, "And this here, this is made of real California redwood."

I couldn't believe my ears at first, and I stood there kind of stunned for a second or two. I didn't want to offend my friend or anything by getting into an argument with his new landlord, but I just had to say something.

"Well, you know," I said, "there's not a lot of that redwood left. As a matter of fact, they're cutting it down at quite a pace and there's only about three per cent of the original old-growth redwoods still standing."

He jumped down off the stage and looked me right in the eye and said, "I know, isn't that terrible?" Then, turning away, he just went on with the tour: "But look at this, see these ceramic tiles over here? These come from Italy . . ."

I guess I could have gotten into it with him, but the damage was already done. It was just a perfect example, though, of how so many of us live our lives isolated from the planet. That guy was just so proud of his nice bar that he didn't make the connection between the redwoods disappearing and his part in that.

The sad thing is, there's nothing unique about that guy in New York; we all do it to some extent. As the dominant species on this planet, the human race has developed a real culture of entitlement, as if everything on earth was put here just for us to use any way we want. We're spoiled, if you want to know the truth, especially in the developed world, and the United States in particular.

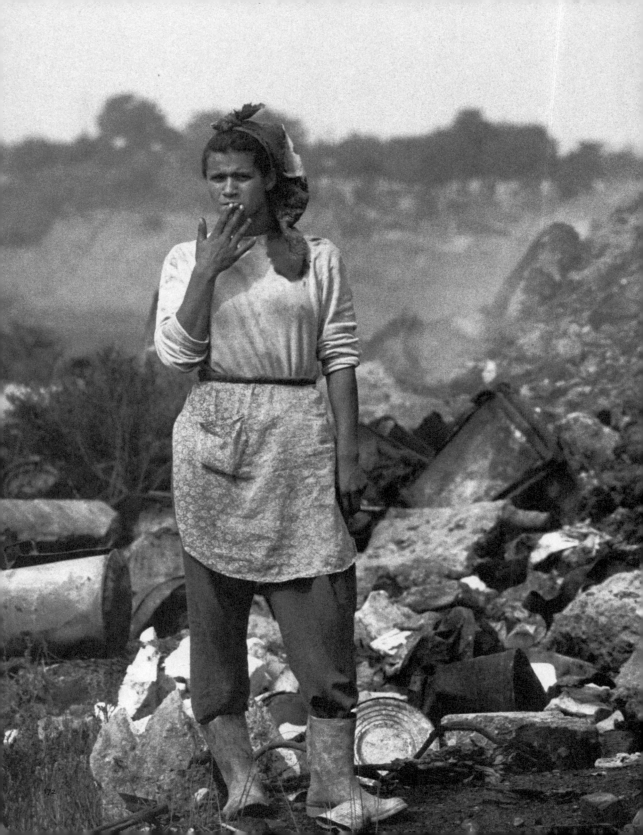

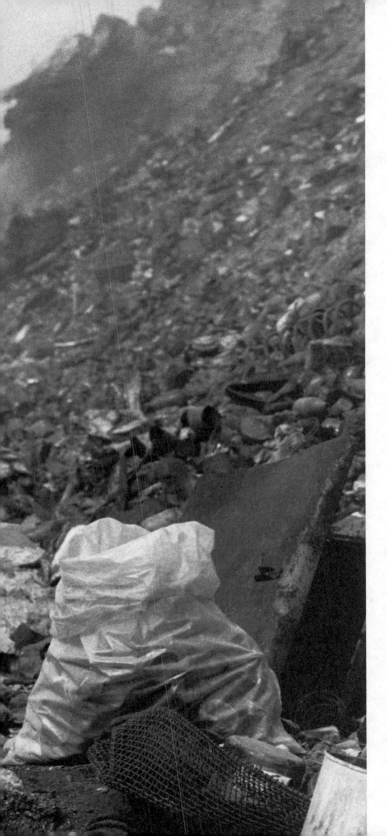

In fact, the environment in the rest of the world is actually subsidizing America's gluttonous appetite for things like oil, paper, meat, cotton, and sugar. But we don't see the environmental damage our appetites cause in other countries, so we don't care. It's like most people don't spend a lot of time wondering whether or not that Nike shirt they love so much was made in some sweatshop in Southeast Asia. Even when it's right under our nose we still find a way to avoid the truth. The logging companies leave a strip of trees standing between the road and acres of clear-cut so we don't have to look at it when we drive by. Cities put the garbage dump on the other side of the tracks, or in the next county, or even ship the garbage out of state so somebody else can deal with it.

And as we're pumping that Premium into the SUV, in the back of our minds we just keep telling ourselves, "Hey, the world's a big place; Mother Nature will survive. There might be a few less redwood trees and a few less species, but she'll survive." But in our heart we know that that's just not the right way to go.

So the question is, how do we start to make those connections? The first thing you have to do is figure out how the things you do in your everyday life are helping the Beast to rape your Mother, because if you're anything like me, you don't want to serve the Beast anymore, and you don't want the Beast serving you.

For me, the connections between my actions and the health of the planet were always there, it just took me a while to start seeing them. I remember when I was sixteen I worked at a church camp in Zanesfield, Ohio, and they gave me a job cleaning the toilets. They gave me this

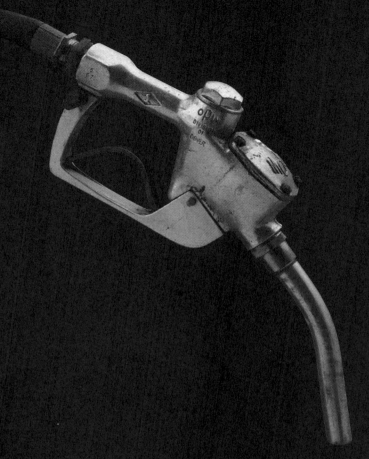

Worldwide:
• The burning
of fossil fuels
has almost quin-
tupled since 1950.
• Fresh water con-
sumption has almost
doubled since 1960.
• Wood consumption rose
40% between 1973 and 1998.
• Annual carbon dioxide emissions havequadrupled since 1950.
• One child born in the industrialized
world adds more to consumption in
his or her lifetime than do 30 to 40 children born in developing countries.
• In industrial countries, waste generated per
capita increased almost threefold in the last two
decades of the 20th century.

Source: Human Devlopment Report 1998 (United Nations Development
Programme, 1998), p. 2.

really powerful industrial cleanser to do it, and one time I accidentally squirted some on my leg. Well, my skin turned red and it stung like hell almost right away, then the hair on that spot on my leg fell off. It stayed that way for about two weeks before it started to go back to normal, but the hair never did grow back. It wasn't until years later though that I thought, "What the hell was in that shit?" It must have been ten times as toxic as whatever I was trying to clean off the toilets.

When you start to look for it, you begin to see the mark of the Beast everywhere. Just look at the number of paper napkins and plastic cups used on your average airplane flight; garbage bags–full are taken off at the end.

That's how it works—it's noticing little things like paper napkins on a plane that helps you make the connections you need to make. You don't just see the napkin going in the trash anymore, you start to think about how many trees are cut down just to make the napkins in the first place, and all the energy that went into manufacturing them and transporting them around. Then there are the chemicals that bleach the paper white, and the ink for the airline logo. What's that shit made of? Does it have petroleum products in it? Are airline napkins really the best use for our precious natural resources, and would gas be twenty-five cents less a gallon if we didn't waste so much crude oil on chemicals and ink and shipping around products that we end up throwing away in brand new condition anyway?

Waste is everywhere in our disposable world, and that's the Beast feeding on our planet. I walked into a café in San Francisco one time and I noticed that every single person sitting in the place—there was about ten of them—had a little paper bag with the company logo on it that their sandwich came in. So every customer in there got their food in a bag so they could go and eat it eight feet away.

Now the people working in the place put the food in the bags because I guess that was the company policy; every sandwich—here you go; here you go; here you go. And the customers, I guess, just took the bags without thinking, because that's what most of us do. But how hard would it be for that café to post a sign that said, "We will gladly give you a bag if you request one, and we ask that you please recycle it if possible"? The company would end up spending a hell of a lot less money on bags, for one thing. Then the owners could take more profit, or pay their employees more, or maybe invest it in better ingredients or equipment or whatever. On top of that, just by showing some concern for the environment, all of a sudden they're "eco-friendly," and they can maybe use that "green" image to attract a whole new group of customers who give a shit about the planet.

So the bottom line is, if you want to stop feeding the Beast, you can start by becoming a conscious consumer. Look at the products you use. Do you have polyester or nylon clothes? They're made from petroleum and that's a mark of the Beast. Do you drink lots of soda? That's refined sugar—mark of the Beast. Do you use Tide or Clorox to wash your clothes? Cascade to wash your dishes? Many detergents contain phosphates, chlorine, and other harmful chemicals that end up in the water system. If you're thinking of buying something made of plastic, you've got to try to keep a few facts in mind: first, plastic is a petroleum product, and we are in an oil war era; second, plastic is not biodegradable, so if it ends up in a landfill after you're finished with it, it's going to be there for the next 500 years.

Being a conscious consumer means reading the ingredients on packages and avoiding the nasty stuff. It means finding out which manufacturers manufacture what, and avoiding the ones that exploit workers and damage the environment. It means making a real effort to look for alternatives, in ingredients, in packaging, even in where you shop and who you buy from.

The real key to saving the earth is refusing to think about things in isolation from one another and instead making the connection between what you do and where you live. It's about disrupting the negative consumption patterns we've been living with for so long. Personal transformation really does equal planetary transformation, because, whether you're aware of it or not, once you change your own behavior and start living a sustainable lifestyle, you become a really powerful role model for others.

Behavioral scientists did a study on "modeling" one time at UC Santa Cruz in California where they put up a

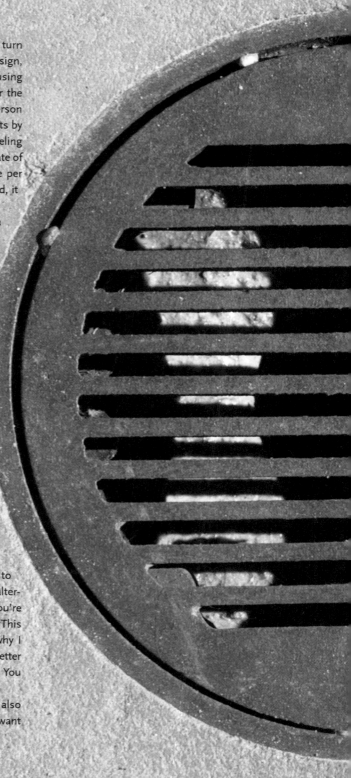

sign in the showers at the gym that read, "Please turn off the shower while soaping up." With just the sign, they found that only nineteen per cent of the guys using the shower turned the water off as requested. For the next stage of the experiment, they put a second person in the shower to act as a role model for the subjects by obeying the sign. With someone else there modeling the correct behavior, the scientists found that the rate of people doing the right thing jumped to forty-nine per cent. When another positive role model was added, it jumped to sixty-seven per cent.

So when you transform your life and become a role model of sustainability for your family and friends, you have a greater impact on the planet than you could possibly know. I'm telling you, it changes people, and it's an exponential change because the circle just keeps getting wider and wider. Just think, if you manage to get three people you know to switch to organic, then they each get three more to switch, it will just keep growing.

So start with yourself. That's not only the best way to change the planet; it's the *only* way. Just like that sign in the shower, you're never going to get anywhere by telling people what they should be doing—it's the whole "holier than thou" thing that people just naturally resist. In fact, if there's anything most people hate it's being told, "Hey man, you're doing that wrong; this is the right way." And that's something I know a lot about, because I spent most of the first half of my life in churches hearing exactly that.

I find it's far more effective to just do your best to live a sustainable life and in that way offer people alternatives. That way, when people ask you what you're doing, you can come at it from a place that says, "This is just another way of doing things, and this is why I think it's a better way...." And that's a hell of a lot better than saying, "This is the way you have to do it." You open up a dialogue without being confrontational.

I believe that most people are smart, and I also believe that most people are essentially good and want

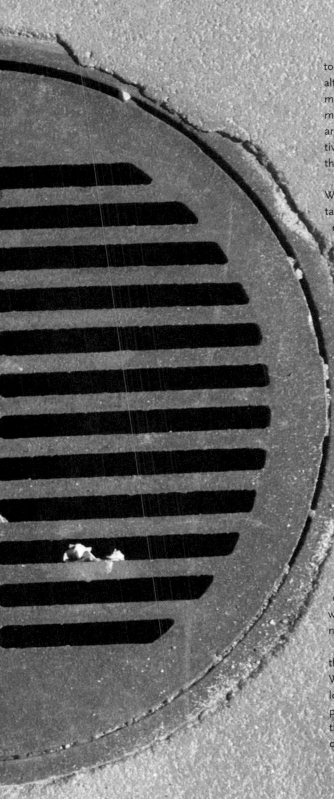

to do the right thing. If you make people aware of the alternatives and give them the information they need to make good choices, I truly believe most people will make the sustainable choice in the end. But if people are never exposed to alternative products and alternative behaviors, we can't expect them to make choices that are better for them and better for the planet.

So at the end of the day, you have to ask yourself: Whose responsibility is it to make people aware of sustainable alternatives? Well, if you live on the same planet I do, I'd say it's *our* responsibility—yours and mine, as individuals and collectively. That's what the SOL Tour was all about: taking responsibility for yourself and the planet; getting out and being a living breathing example of simple organic living.

And if you're ever looking for motivation, just look into the eyes of a child for a while; that always does it for me. You know, my generation, people born in the 1960s, we've been lucky enough to see a living redwood tree and gray whales breaching off the coast of California, but that's only because people stood up in the 1960s and started the environmental movement.

Now it's our turn, and if we start now, we have a good chance of saving something for future generations. I'm happy my kids have been able to see a redwood tree and a California gray whale, but I want my grandkids to see those things too, and their grandkids after that. Our parents and grandparents messed things up pretty bad, but they didn't really know what we know now and they didn't have the technology we have today. The fact is, we could fuck things up worse today than they ever could have imagined if we're not careful.

I don't know about anybody else but I don't want that on my conscience twenty or thirty years from now. What kind of legacy would it be if future generations look back and say, "I can't believe how my grandparents poisoned the earth, air and water. Now fifty per cent of their descendants get cancer; half of their descendants die before they turn fifty." That's what inspires me to try

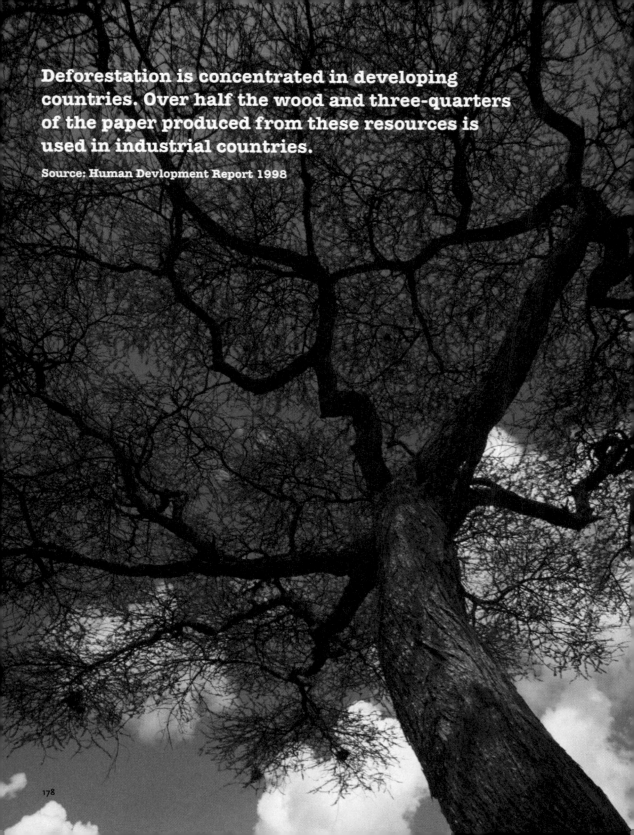

Deforestation is concentrated in developing countries. Over half the wood and three-quarters of the paper produced from these resources is used in industrial countries.

Source: Human Devlopment Report 1998

The percentage of Americans describing themselves as happy peaked in 1957—even though consumption has doubled since then.

Source: Human Devlopment Report 1998

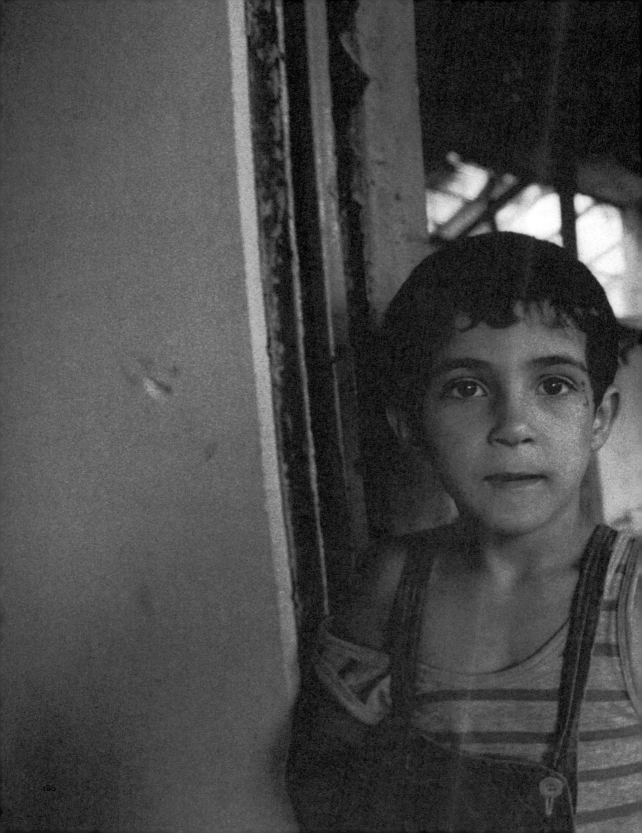

...to make a difference, I want my grandkids to know I did the best I could for them.

The best possible legacy we could leave for our kids and grandkids is a sustainable way of living that they learn from watching us practice it. If we can relearn all the things our parents took for granted, like where we get our resources, what we use for energy, what we buy at the grocery store, we can save our kids the trouble of doing the same thing down the road. If we make the effort to break those negative patterns now, then maybe it won't become such a pathology for future generations.

It takes courage to break those old patterns, and there are lots of people who have a vested interest in keeping us on the wrong path. But I think any time you stand up for anything there's going to be somebody who doesn't stand for the same thing, so there's always a risk there. But I also believe that when what you're doing is right, you'll turn on twice as many people as you turn off and the circle will grow.

A change is coming, one way or another. And, one way or another, people who don't change are going to get Wookied. It may be happening slowly, but we're in the middle of a giant mass extinction on our planet, and we're the cause. Now we have to decide if we're going to be a species that gets extinguished just like all the others we've helped along.

Personal transformation equals planetary transformation—it's a revolution that starts with one person. You can do it. We have to—our Mother is depending on us.

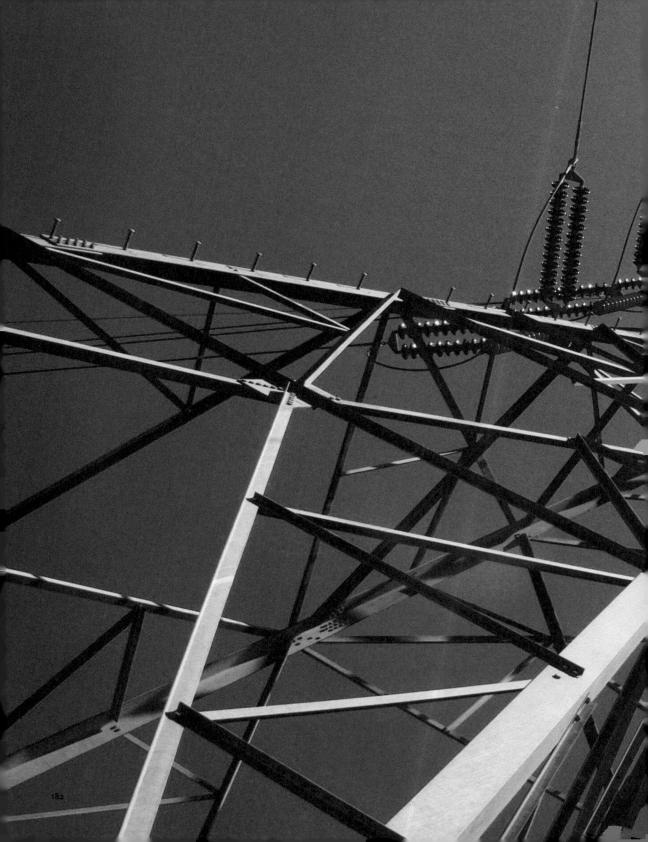

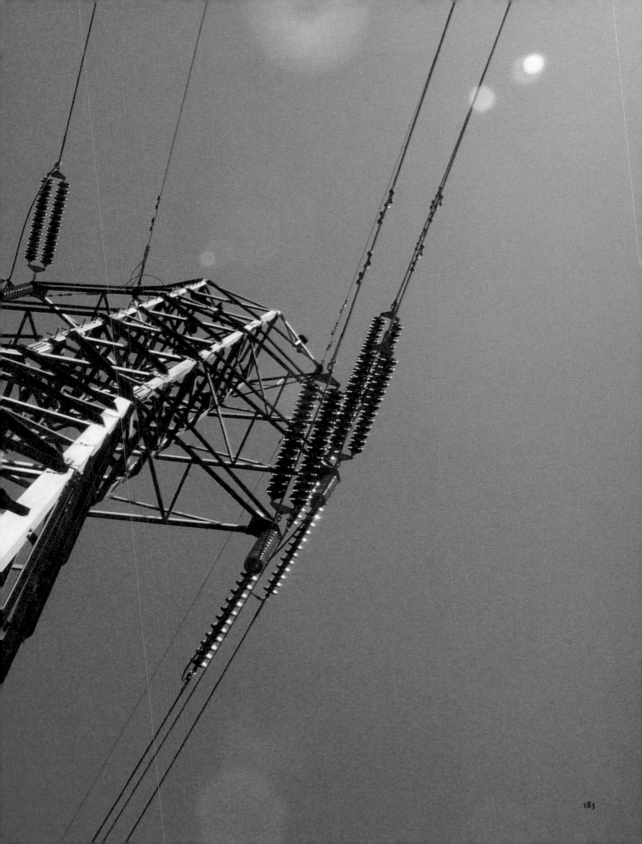

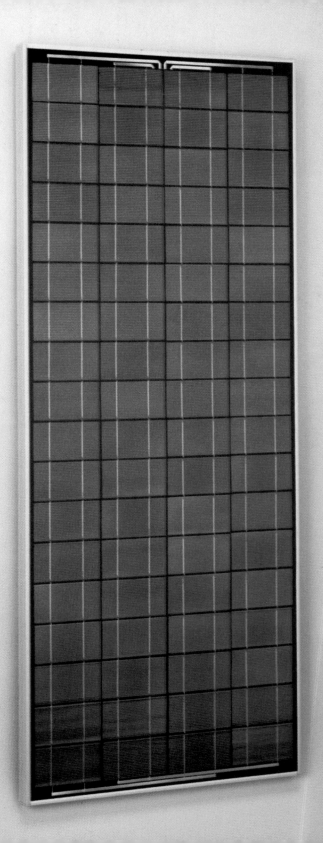

ALTERNATIVE ENERGY

John Schaeffer

If you are familiar with the name Enron, you probably know that an energy meltdown has occurred in California and the western United States in the last few years. On the heels of California's ill-conceived 1996 deregulation scheme, out-of-state utilities cashed in on an energy scarcity opportunity, increasing prices for electricity and natural gas as much as six-fold. That sure got a lot of people thinking about where their power comes from and how much it costs to produce. From my perspective, though, the collapse of the deregulated power market is not a new, or unexpected turn of events. In fact, before long the entire country will be coping with the same forces that are shaping California's energy crisis.

In the summer of 2003, we received another wake-up call as a large portion of the eastern U.S. and Canada lost power. Before long, politicians everywhere were grandstanding, using the blackout to justify all kinds of bizarre agendas. I even heard Sean Hannity of *Fox News* claiming that the blackout was the result of our failure to drill oil in Alaska. In a country as short-sighted as the United State, it takes the image of tens of thousands of people walking lock-step across the Brooklyn Bridge and a blacked-out Times Square to get people's attention.

The simple fact is that it's not just our electric system that is creaky, outmoded, and nearly obsolete but also the entire underlying Industrial Age paradigm of centralized power. Clearly, the world needs to come to its senses and eliminate its dependence upon fossil fuels. And, as we move through the early days of the third millennium, it is becoming increasingly clear that the era of oil and fossil fuels is coming to an end. We sit on the cusp of a new paradigm. Behind us (we hope) is the wanton devastation and destruction of natural habitat, while before us is the bountiful opportunity for a fruitful and fulfilling future. But we have to play our cards correctly, and this means understanding our finite energy resources.

From society's standpoint, the stage is already set for a rapid conversion from an economy based on fossil fuel energy to one based on renewable energy. However, obstructionist policies by entrenched political and business interests threaten to block that conversion and engulf our planet in a deathly haze of greenhouse gases. Whether we have the foresight to take heed of our natural limits or continue our unfettered consumption becomes the ultimate question for our species. Our fate is in our own hands.

In our favor is the fact that ours is the first generation in history to know that we are in danger of self-destruction. At least we should; the signs are everywhere:

Fresh water is scarce. Worldwide water use has tripled since 1950, resulting in huge water deficits in key river basins in China and India. In India, with its one billion inhabitants, the extraction of water from aquifers is twice its annual recharge. What will happen when the population grows by an expected 600 million by 2050?

We have exceeded the sustainable yield of oceanic fisheries. Eleven of the world's fifteen most important fishing areas and seventy per cent of the major fish species are either depleted or overexploited.

The world's forests face similar devastation. Nearly half of the forests that once covered the earth are gone. In just fifteen years, between 1980 and 1995, more than 400 million acres—an area larger than all of Mexico—were lost. And the rate of forest destruction is accelerating.

But the number one indicator of the earth's failing health is the shrinking number of plant and animal species. Of 242,000 plant species on the planet, fourteen per cent or 33,000 are threatened because of habitat destruction. Of 9,600 bird species in existence, sixty-seven per cent are in decline and eleven per cent are facing extinction. The outlook for fish and mammals is equally bleak.

Our legacy from the era of oil and fossil fuels is global warming. Carbon emissions exceed the capacity of the earth's natural systems to "fix" carbon dioxide. Since scientists began recording average annual earth temperatures in 1866, the sixteen warmest years on record have all occurred since 1980. The year 1998 was the warmest on record, and also represented the

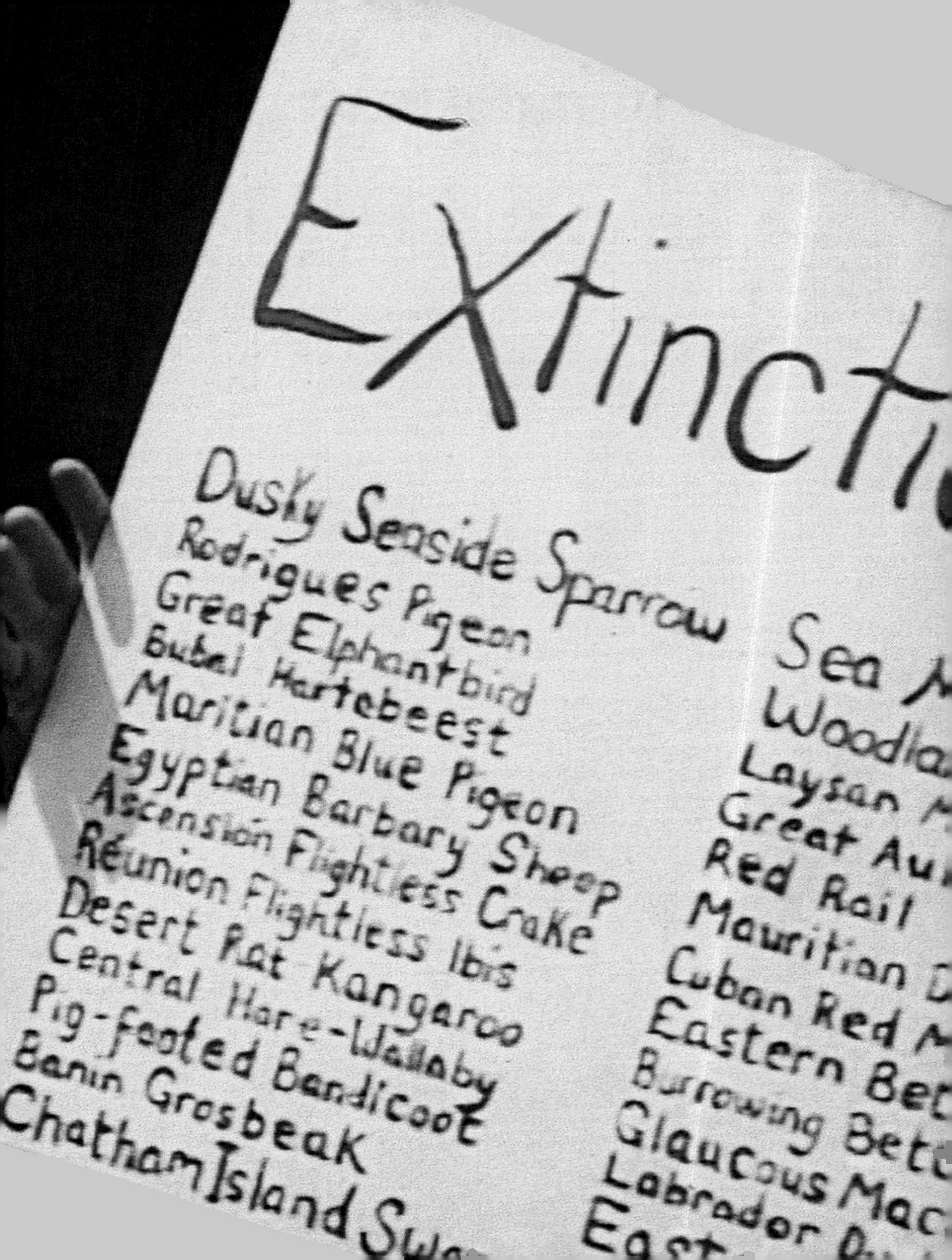

Extincti

Dusky Seaside Sparrow Sea
Rodrigues Pigeon
Great Elephantbird
Bubal Hartebeest
Maritian Blue Pigeon
Egyptian Barbary Sheep
Ascension Flightless Crake
Réunion Flightless Ibis
Desert Rat Kangaroo
Central Hare-Wallaby
Pig-footed Bandicoot
Benin Grosbeak
Chatham Island Swa

Woodla
Laysan
Great Au
Red Rail
Mauritian
Cuban Red
Eastern Bet
Burrowing Bett
Glaucous Mac
Labrador D
East

largest-ever single-year increase. The impact of unchecked global warming is the stuff of a Hollywood disaster movie, with oceans expected to rise an estimated three to ten inches in the next century. Moreover, the impact on other species will likely be more devastating than that on humans.

The U.S. Congress's own Office of Technology Assessment estimates that all known oil reserves will have been depleted by 2037. And yet, the playing field remains tilted in favor of the entrenched oil interests. Over $100 billion in subsidies are available to the fossil fuel industry, while incentives for renewable energy sources are minimal. Obviously, there are strong factions who have a vested interest in maintaining the sta-tus quo. In the 1996 election, oil and gas companies gave $11.8 million to congressional candidates in order to protect tax breaks worth at least $3 billion. George W. Bush makes no secret of his ties to big oil, nor the extent of contributions received from it during his campaign. The powers of entrenchment are indeed formidable.

But there is hope: the revolution is occurring at the grassroots level where there has been a blossoming of many "cultural creative" pursuits. Sales of organic food, for example, grew nineteen-fold from $180 million in 1980 to $3.5 billion in 1996. The same kind of paradigm shift can be seen with the 2001 energy "crisis," which we prefer to call a giant energy "opportunity." Another hopeful sign is the new renewable energy

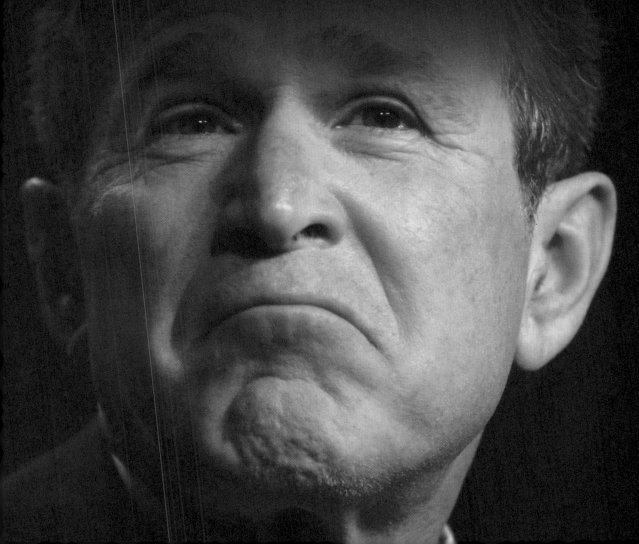

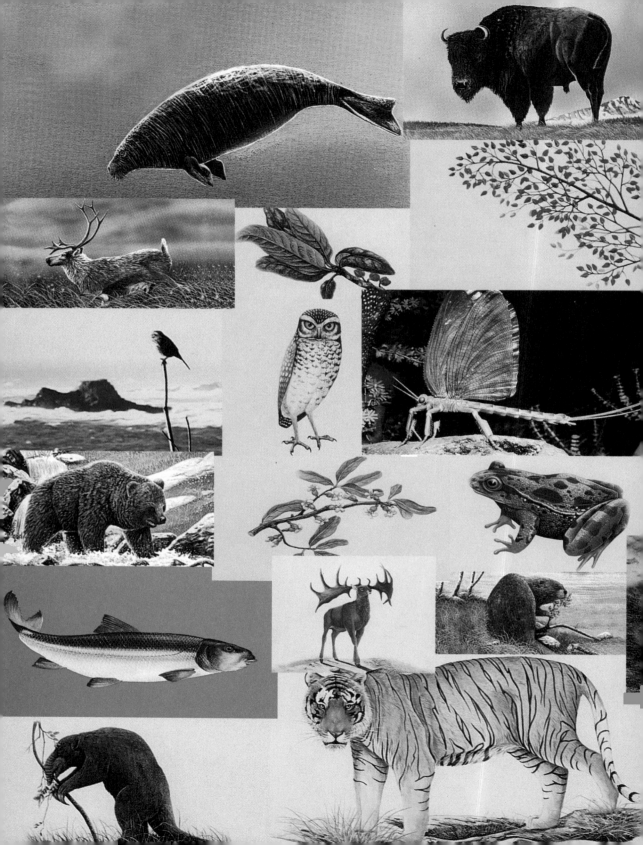

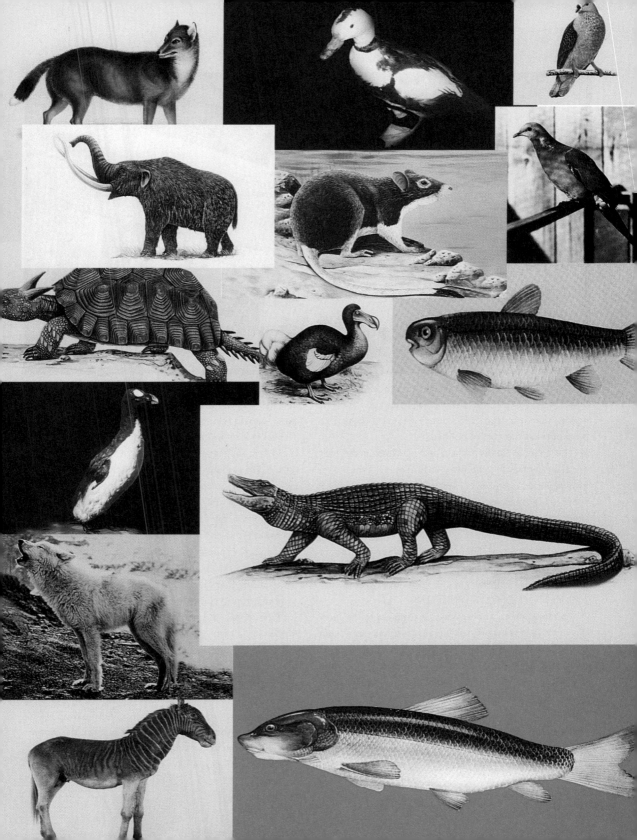

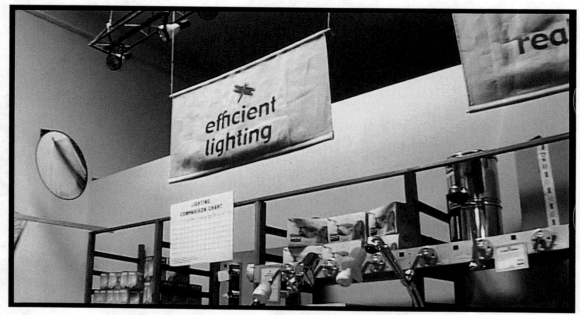

buydown programs that have been introduced at the state level. People are getting the message. Now it seems the only true "blackouts" are the intelligence blackouts on the part of politicians.

The crisis in California and the blackout in the east are clear signals that we need to fundamentally change how America designs its electricity system so that it's more reliable and more resilient. The solution is distributed generation—placing smaller, modular, diverse, and redundant electrical devices across the grid close to the loads they serve. Energy sources like photovoltaics (PV), fuel cells, and micro-hydro can provide power at lower cost and with far greater reliability than the centralized power grid.

At a time when innocent people continue to die every day in a relentless war for oil in Iraq, there has never been a greater need to demonstrate that renewable energy is abundant, practical, economical, clean, and safe. When our company, Real Goods, sold the first retail photovoltaic module in America in 1978 for over $100 per watt, little did we expect that twenty-five years later over five million of those same PV modules would be sold annually, and that the price would have decreased twenty-fold to make it affordable and one of the best investments in

America. And solar provides maximum power just when it's needed—in the middle of the summer afternoon, when air conditioning loads are heaviest and a huge bottleneck occurs in transmission lines.

There are signs that alternative sources like solar power are gaining acceptance. Federal, state, and local governments are now subsidizing renewables through manufacturer and end-user rebates. In California, the California Energy Commission (CEC) enables us to sell renewable power for fifty per cent less than retail price. And San Francisco, Alameda County, and the Sacramento Municipal Utilities District are strongly considering huge PV arrays to keep their municipalities running during summer blackouts.

Best of all, the cost of getting off the grid keeps declining. With the price of installed solar now approaching three to four dollars per watt (after a fifty per cent state rebate), the payback period is five to ten years with a guaranteed price of $0.09/kWh for the next thirty years. That amounts to a ten to twenty per cent return on investment. With utilities now paying up to $0.40/kWh, the return on investment for the homeowner is now approaching what it was for dot-com stocks in the halcyon days of the NASDAQ.

All around the world, there are signs that the stage is set for positive change. While the use of coal, oil, and nuclear power during the 1990s expanded by only slightly more than one per cent each annually, the use of photovoltaics has grown by seventeen per cent annually and wind-generated electricity by twenty-six per cent. While there are still two billion people in the world without access to electricity (and another billion who have it less than ten hours per day), there are now 500,000 homes worldwide (mostly in Third World villages) powered by photovoltaics. Maybe they know something that we don't know—that power from the sun is the best power you can get.

I believe we are on the brink of a major change in consciousness. But whether the scales will tip toward exceeding our natural limits or proactively managing our fate is still unknown. We know our species can't survive the continued loss of bio-diversity, the decimation of forests, the shrinking of ocean fisheries, and the fouling of our atmosphere. We simply have to make things right. It is not too late to build a society that is environmentally sustainable, where water is safe to drink, air is safe to breathe, and communities, even countries, share resources equitably. Let us work toward a future where our great-grandchildren can look back and say, "Thank goodness they finally came to their senses."

John Schaeffer is the founder and president of Real Goods. On its twelve-acre demonstration site in Hopland, California, the company operates a Solar Living Center, a Renewable Energy Division, and a non-profit Solar Living Institute, which provides education and inspirational solutions to our "beyond-the-limits" predicament.

The entire Real Goods site is fully powered by wind and solar energy and demonstrates permaculture, sustainability, and ecological building practices. In the summer of 2003, Real Goods added a new organic farm component, a bio-diesel fueling station, housing for interns, and there are plans to erect a ten-kW Jacobs wind generator at the site. Each August, Real Goods welcomes nearly 200,000 visitors to its annual SolFest celebration, where it presents some of the seminal thinkers of our time in the area of sustainable living. If you'd like to support the non-profit Institute, please consider a donation or becoming a partner (Telephone: 707-744-2017; website: www.realgoods.com).

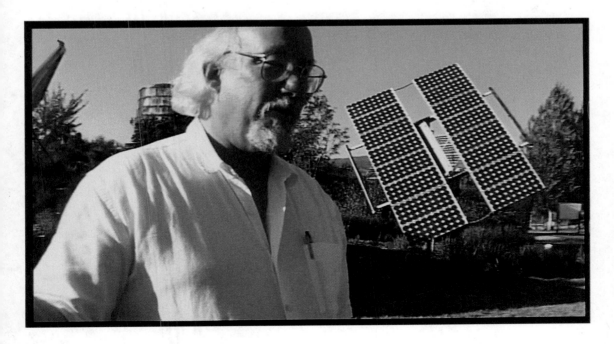

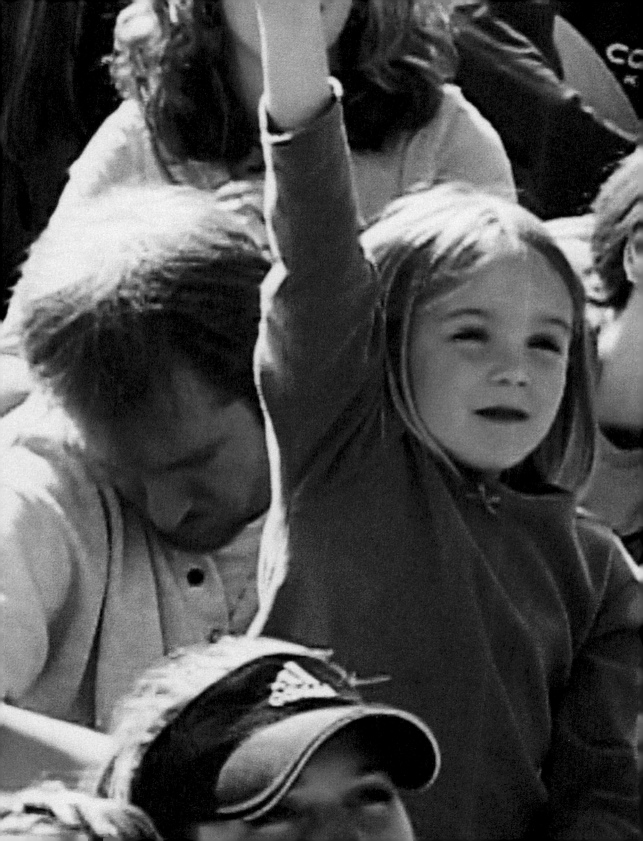

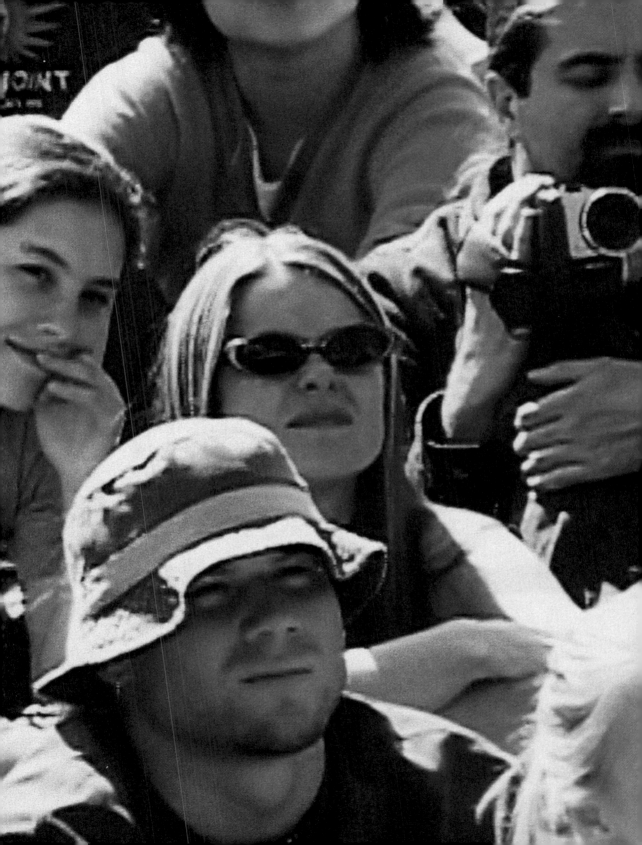

THE BALLAD OF JOE HICKEY:
An Activist is Born

Joe Hickey

I think all of us have times when we stop to look around at where life has taken us and we just have to ask ourselves, "How the hell did I get here?"

One of those times came for me in May 2001; that's when I found myself riding a bike through a grove of hundred-foot redwood trees in Northern California next to a guy I'd been watching on TV and in movies for years. The guy was Woody Harrelson, who by that time had become a very dear friend of mine, and we happened to be in Northern California because we were in the middle of a little bike trip we were taking down the West Coast.

The SOL Tour was just a happy band of people trav-eling around and spreading the word about eating right,

living right, and saving the planet, and I was one of them. It sure was a long way from home for an old Kentucky farm boy like me, and I have to admit, I asked myself what the hell I was doing there more than once—usually five or six times a day at least.

Of all the people who took part in the SOL Tour, I think I probably took the most unlikely route to get there. I wasn't a member of Woody's family, first of all, and I didn't work in show business. I also can't say I qualify as an expert on "alternative" lifestyles, and I don't think anybody would ever confuse me with a hip-pie. I did know a thing or two about fighting for worth-while causes though, so I guess Woody figured he'd like an old protest buddy along for the ride in case the going got rough. After all, that's what brought Woody and me together and made us friends in the first place.

• • •

I was born into a family of nine kids in the small town of Lebanon, Kentucky. The area around had all kinds of farms—cattle, grain, and lots of tobacco; tobacco was the big cash crop in Kentucky back in those days.

My family ran a funeral home, but funeral homes and kids don't mix, so usually, whenever there was a funeral, we got sent off to my grandfather's farm for the day, and that's where I spent most of my spare time as a kid.

After high school I got into construction and eventually started my own business in Lexington, Kentucky, doing commercial renovations. In the late 1980s, when the work dried up in Lexington, we moved our operation down to Belize and built things for the government there for a couple of years. Then the government changed on us and we lost all our contracts, so I came back to Kentucky.

At that point, I had had just about enough of the construction business, so I took a little hiatus from work, just to spend time reading and fixing things up around the house.

My dad had died in early 1989, and one day, when I was going through some of his things, I came upon a bunch of old issues of the *Lexington Herald* newspaper. I started to flip through them and found the history fascinating. I got to read first-hand accounts of Charles Lindbergh's flight, the rise of Hitler in the 1930s, and the front in World War Two. Then, while reading a paper from 1943, I came upon a story headlined, "F.G. Clay resigns from the Kentucky Hemp Growers Co-op."

The article was about how President Roosevelt had asked this F.G. Clay to come to Washington during WWII to run something called the "Hemp for Victory" program. Now that really grabbed my attention, if for no other reason than it sounded so funny. I knew there was a difference between hemp and marijuana, but back in the early '90s, if you said "hemp" to most people, probably ninety-nine per cent would think you were talking about pot. Anyway, the newspaper article made it clear that the association had existed back then, and I found that really intriguing.

The next day, I drove to the state capitol to see if there was any official record of this Kentucky Hemp Growers Co-operative. Lo and behold, a search of the state archives yielded a whole mass of documents. Probably the most interesting among them were the original incorporation papers for the Co-op, which included the names of the twenty original members of the board of directors. I found out later that these board members were a who's who of the Kentucky agricultural community at that time. One was listed as a bank executive acting on behalf of the Bank of Versailles, a prominent bank in Kentucky. All this just amazed me—here were the most distinguished men in the state in the 1940s, plus a well-established bank, all actively involved in producing a crop that is just about Public Enemy Number One today.

I couldn't let it drop after that; I had to find out why the hemp industry in my home state had simply vanished. I didn't know exactly what I was going to do with this information. I guess it was a bit like quicksand: you start by putting one foot in, and before you know it you're neck-deep in it.

No matter how you look at it, it was weird. I did more research and found out that hemp was basically made illegal by the federal government in 1937 through something called the Marijuana Tax Act, but the incorporation papers said that the original Kentucky Hemp Growers Co-operative was formed in 1941. And the tax records showed that the co-operative was running right up until some time in 1947, when it basically disappeared. So apparently, at the urging of the federal government, the Kentucky hemp industry was pulled out of mothballs by these prominent members of the agricultural community to help the war effort, and local farmers were encouraged to grow hemp again after being told not to just a few years before. I even found a 4-H flyer encouraging teenage farmers to plant an acre of hemp for seed. I just about fell over when I saw that—the government encouraging "the farmers of tomorrow" to grow hemp.

I found out from the state historical board that there were seventeen historical markers around Kentucky that actually mentioned hemp. So I drove around looking for

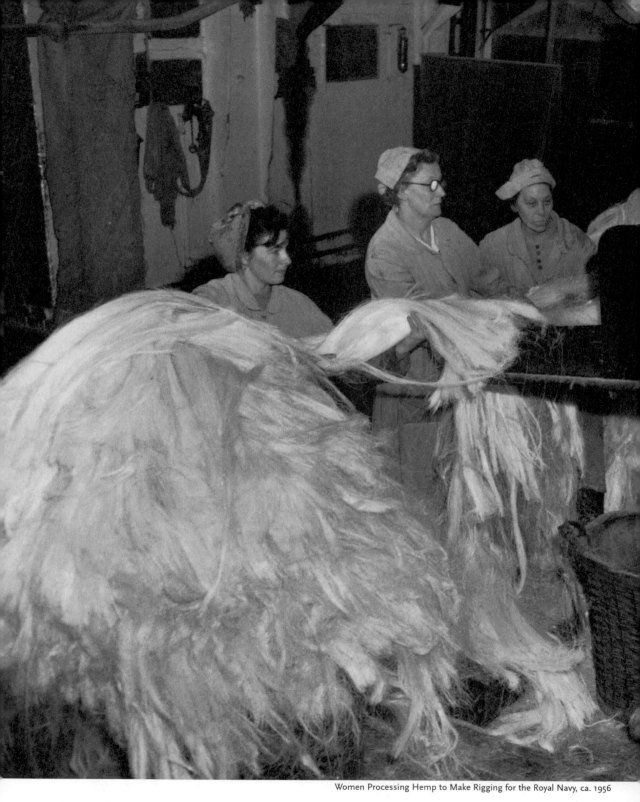

Women Processing Hemp to Make Rigging for the Royal Navy, ca. 1956

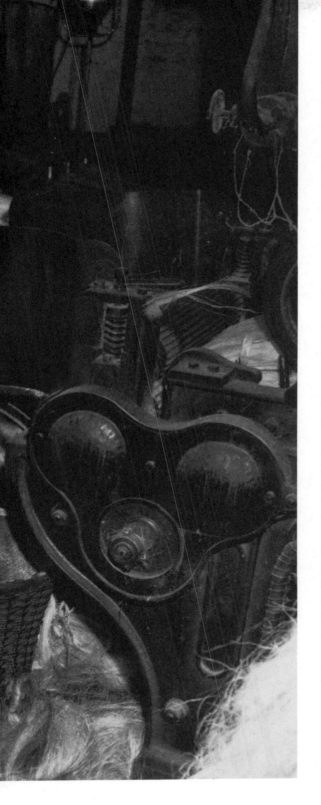

these markers and taking pictures of them. They turned out to be typical historical plaques—some in the center of small towns or on old warehouses and factories—and they mentioned things like how much hemp was grown in the area, how many feet of rope was manufactured for the war effort, and how much money the hemp industry generated for the state.

I contacted a man named James Hopkins, who had written a book entitled, *The History of Hemp in Kentucky*. He told me about a place called Woodford Feed in Paris, Kentucky, that used to be a hemp processing facility. So off I went to Paris and, sure enough, they still had the old grinding stones and various machines used for processing the hemp fiber.

The guy running the place let me in to this dusty old back office and in a couple of battered filing cabinets I found an absolute treasure trove of information about the Kentucky hemp industry going back almost one hundred years. There were records of who was growing hemp, how much they were growing, letters from the War Department, letters from the Navy—it took me days to go through it all.

I also took some of the hemp fiber that was still lying on the floor under the old machines. My wife and I got one of those little paper-making kits that kids use and we made several sheets of paper using the hemp fibers. We were amazed because it came out looking just like the paper the Bible is printed on.

But around this time my hemp research kind of stalled. I had collected all this evidence but I still wasn't sure what the heck I was going to do with it. I could easily prove that there had been a thriving hemp industry in Kentucky prior to and during the Second World War, but so what? At that point, you could say I was all dressed up with nowhere to go.

Then a tobacco farmer friend told me that Kimberley-Clark, the huge multinational consumer goods company, was making cigarette paper and paper for Bibles out of hemp over in France, where it is legal to grow it. Well, I got right on the phone to the French embassy in Washington and, about ten calls later, finally got directed to the "Department of Hemp" at the French Ministry of Agriculture in Paris, France. (That really made me laugh—

in the U.S. you go to jail for growing hemp, and in France they have a government department devoted to it.)

I was put through to an English-speaking staff member who told me they had been growing hemp, or *chanvre*, commercially in France for literally hundreds of years and nobody ever had a problem with it as far as he knew. He also gave me the phone number of a guy in England named Ian Lowe who was petitioning the government there to allow the commercial production of hemp in that country.

I called Ian up and he turned out to be a really nice, helpful guy. I told him my story and we were on the same wavelength right away because we were both old country boys. He sold farm supplies, so he was right up on all the laws pertaining to agriculture in Britain. He told me how he had applied to the British Home Office—which is like the U.S. State Department—for a permit to grow industrial hemp under the rules governing the European Union, and he was sure they were going to give it to him.

He put me in contact with a guy in Canada named Joe Strobble who was applying to the Canadian government for a permit to grow hemp there. Joe, who, ironically enough, was a tobacco farmer, was just as confident as Ian that he was going to get his permit as well, and was already planning a hemp crop for the next growing season.

All this led me to consider hemp as an alternative cash crop for Kentucky tobacco farmers. This was around the time that the anti-smoking movement was really gathering momentum and it looked like the days of tobacco ruling the roost in Kentucky would be coming to an end soon. I finally knew what to do with all the information I'd collected: I was going to try to make it legal for farmers to grow industrial hemp again in Kentucky. The only question was, how was I going to do it?

Then, right on cue, another one of life's crazy coincidences moved me a little farther down the track. I don't listen to the radio much, but one day I happened to be sitting in the kitchen with the radio on and I heard about something that the governor at the time, Brereton Jones, was doing called "Open Doors After Four." The way it worked was, one afternoon a month after 4:00,

any resident of the state could show up at the governor's office and have a private audience with him for ten or fifteen minutes to talk about any subject that was important to him or her. Now I knew what my next step would be.

I called the governor's office and signed up for the After Four program. When the day came, my wife and I drove over to the governor's office early in the afternoon and waited. Eventually, we were ushered into a big paneled room where we were interviewed by the governor's executive assistant. He asked us about everything— where we were from, where we went to school, what we did for a living, what we did in our spare time, and finally, what we wanted to talk to the governor about. As I was getting grilled, I started to think that maybe it wouldn't be such a good idea to tell this guy that I wanted to talk about the possibility of growing hemp for profit. So when he asked me what I wanted to talk about, I said I wanted to discuss "ways to avert the crisis Kentucky farmers face with the looming downturn in the tobacco industry."

That must have been good enough for him, because he just stood up and said, "All right, if you'll follow me, I'll take you down to the governor's office."

We followed him down a long hallway to a huge office where Governor Jones was sitting behind the desk. We shook hands, then the governor glanced at a piece of paper the assistant had handed him and said to me, "OK Mr. Hickey, what's your solution to the tobacco problem?"

I have to admit, I was more than a little nervous but I figured there was no turning back at that point. So I swallowed hard and said: "Well Governor, I guess you probably know that it's an historical fact that we grew industrial hemp in Kentucky right up until just after World War II. It's legal for farmers to grow it in France right now, and they're getting ready to make it legal for farmers to grow it in England and Canada, so I think it's a cash crop that we should give serious consideration to in Kentucky. There are all kinds of uses for industrial hemp, and it could be a great alternative if tobacco farmers have to start cutting down on their tobacco acreage in the future."

When I finished my little speech, the governor just sat back in his chair and gave me that look people always give you when you utter the word "hemp"—the kind that says, "Oh my God, not one of these hippie freaks."

So we all sat there for a few seconds with nobody saying anything; I was sure that at any moment some security guy was going to put his hand on my shoulder and say, "OK Hickey, out you go." But that didn't happen. The governor rocked back in his chair and you could see he was rolling what I said over in his mind. Finally, he looked at the stack of papers I was holding in my lap and said, "What have you got there?"

I had brought some documentation with me—photos of the old hemp processing equipment and the historical markers; copies of the incorporation papers from the Kentucky Hemp Growers Co-operative and letters from the War Department; and a list of the regulations governing the production of hemp in the European Union Ian Lowe had sent me. I had also brought a few sheets of the hemp paper we had made at home.

I spread all this stuff out on a table in the office and the governor just stood silently looking at it as I explained to him what each thing was. He went back to his desk and sat down and was quiet for a few minutes, then he said, "If you were me Joe, what would you do with this information you've shown me today?"

"Well Governor," I said, "if it were me, I think I'd want to look into this and see if hemp really can be a viable alternative for Kentucky farmers. I guess I'd probably set up some kind of task force or something to see if we can get our hemp industry going again."

He just nodded and said, "Joe, you're exactly right. I know hemp has a public perception problem, but it's time we all got over that."

Then he looked over at his executive assistant and said, "Jim, could you get Mr. Hickey here together with the right people at the Department of Agriculture and let's get this going."

Well, you could have knocked me over with a feather right then. The most I had expected was some non-committal response like, "Well Joe, we'll take your ideas under advisement."

After that we shook hands and my wife and I were escorted out of the office by one of the governor's bodyguards, a big heavy-set state trooper. As we were walking down the steps of the governor's office, he said to us, "You know, everything you said in there is exactly right; our farmers are going to need something if the tobacco falls off. But you're going to have one big problem getting this off the ground."

"Why's that?" I asked.

"Law enforcement spends an awful lot of time and money fighting drugs in this state, and that's the way it's been for years," he said. "I don't think the powers that be in the law enforcement community are going to stand by and let the legislature make growing hemp legal again."

I really didn't think that much about what he said at the time, but in the ensuing years, that trooper's words came back to me again and again.

Around that time I met up with an old friend named Dave Spalding who worked for the University of Kentucky helping farmers put in new crops. We decided that if the Kentucky hemp industry was ever going to get off the ground again, we were going to need seed. Unlike other cash crops, you can't just go down to the local farm supply and buy a few pounds of hemp seed, so the first task was to create some kind of hemp seed inventory that would be there if and when the legislature ever made it legal to grow again. The only way to do that was to gather seed from wild hemp plants that still grew around the state like weeds, beside back roads and at the ends of farmers' fields.

Dave knew one farmer who had some wild hemp growing on his place, so we went out to see him and he was only too happy to let us have it. "If you don't take it, the cops will just come and cut it down like they do at the end of every year," he said.

That struck Dave and me as kind of funny, so the farmer explained to us how it worked. Apparently, if they cut down the hemp plants earlier on in the summer when they weren't fully grown, they wouldn't "seed out," as the farmers say, and you wouldn't get a new crop the next spring. By waiting until the mature hemp plants go to seed, they're assured that the wild crop will be back the next year and they'll have to come back again to cut that down. It's like an ongoing make-work project for law enforcement.

Now we had our seeds and the task force was moving forward, so things were going pretty good for my little project at that point. That's when I decided it was time to reactivate the Kentucky Hemp Growers Co-operative.

Given the current profile of hemp in the U.S., I knew that we had to get some well-respected members of the Kentucky agricultural community involved if we ever wanted to be taken seriously, and, once again, luck was on my side. Dave Spalding knew a man named Jake Graves who came from a long line of hemp farmers and who had recently retired as chairman of National City Bank in Lexington and had served previously on the Federal Reserve Board. So I went to see Jake, and he graciously agreed to sign on as president of the reconstituted Kentucky Hemp Growers Co-operative. I couldn't have wished for a more dignified, connected, well-respected gentleman farmer to head up our organization. Nobody would think of questioning the motives of a man like that who endorsed industrial hemp.

It took about three months from the time I met with Governor Jones, but he was true to his word and finally announced the task force on industrial hemp. The governor originally wanted our new president, Jake Graves, to head the task force, but Jake refused because he didn't want anyone to think the task force was biased. So the chairman's job went to a guy named Billy Joe Miles, a well-connected businessman from Western Kentucky. I gave Mr. Miles all the information and contacts that I had spent many months collecting so the task force members could get right up to speed on the subject and hurry things along. I shouldn't have bothered.

I was pretty optimistic when it got started, but it didn't take long for me to realize that Billy Joe Miles was in no hurry to see Kentucky farmers growing hemp again. In total, the task force met just three times over the course of five or six months, and by the second meeting you could see Miles wasn't very keen on hemp. At one point I remember Miles saying, "If you guys can find me a Fortune 500 company that's interested in this, then we'll talk." Well, that pretty much told you everything you needed to know about his position on the subject.

Still, we weren't ready to throw in the towel. Just before the task force got started, some of the members of the new co-operative started working with a local cardboard box company called Inland Container to see if they could find an application for hemp. One of the things Inland did was collect old cardboard and mash it up to make new boxes, but they had to add additional wood fiber to the mixture to give the recycled cardboard enough strength. We gave them some hemp fiber to try and they found that the hemp was so strong that they could use much less of it than of the wood fiber in the recycled boxes, which would save them a lot of money. We told Billy Joe Miles about Inland and even tried to set up a meeting with Inland management and the task force, but Billy Joe was just too busy to see anybody.

When the third meeting of the task force got underway, Miles had his assistant pass out a package to each member. When they opened it up they all practically fell out of their chairs. The packages contained nicely printed and bound copies of a publication entitled, "The Final Report of the Governor's Task Force on Hemp."

As everyone sat there stunned, Billy Joe Miles said, "All right ladies and gentlemen, I move that the members of the task force vote to approve this report at this time so we can send it on to the governor's office."

There was no reaction from anybody for a few seconds. Then Gale Glenn, one of the four farmers on the task force spoke up. "Just a minute, Mr. Miles. I'm not going to vote to approve a report I haven't even read. In fact, this is the first time any of us have even seen this report." Jake Graves expressed similar reservations.

Miles basically ignored them and just kept on pushing forward. "Are there any other comments?" he said.

The four farmers on the task force were obviously beside themselves over what was happening, but the other members just sat there in silence. We found out later that that probably had something to do with the fact that Billy Joe Miles sat on the board of governors of the University of Kentucky, and all the other task force members were beholden, in one way or another, to the university.

So Billy Joe just kept asking, "Any more comments?" And finally, when it was obvious the farmers were not going to get any help from the rest of the task force, he put it to a vote.

"All in favor of the report please raise their hand," he said, and everyone but the four farmers raised their hand.

"All opposed?" he said next, and the four farmers put their hands up.

"All right, the motion to approve the final report is carried," said Miles. "As chairman, I now declare the task force dissolved and I thank everyone for their participation."

And that was it. Like Billy Joe Miles, the task force report just blew off the whole issue; it basically said that we didn't know enough about industrial hemp to go ahead at this time and that more study was needed. I don't know if Miles was under pressure from more powerful agriculture interests or if hemp was just a political hot potato, but it was obvious from the way the task force was railroaded that somebody in the state had a big problem with hemp.

The task force was a big disappointment, but it didn't keep us down for long. We started to lobby state legislators to get behind a bill to make it legal for farmers to grow hemp. Lots of them were sympathetic, but they were still pretty leery of the whole idea of hemp. One legislator told me straight: "Look Joe, until you can educate my constituents and convince them that this isn't just some way to legalize pot, I can't support you."

So the Co-operative created the Kentucky Hemp Museum and Library. We traveled around to county fairs, chamber of commerce meetings, and farm bureau meetings to show people the materials and equipment we had collected and to drum up support for reviving the hemp industry. We played videos from Ian Lowe showing European farmers harvesting hemp and some of the things they did with it. We must have been doing something right, because we started to get quite a bit of media coverage.

A year later, in the spring of 1995, I was sitting in the Kentucky Hemp Growers Co-operative office (my bedroom) talking to Jake when the phone rang. My son answered it, and said, "Hey Dad, this guy on the phone says he's Woody Harrelson and he wants to talk to you."

Well, I just laughed—I figured it was one of my friends pulling my leg, but I played along anyway and took the phone.

"Hi Joe, this is Woody Harrelson," said the guy on the other end. "I've been reading about what you guys are doing out there in Kentucky to get the hemp industry going again and I'd love to come out and talk to you about it."

I was always a big *Cheers* fan, and when I heard the voice on the phone I thought to myself, "Man, if that's not Woody Harrelson, it's about the best Woody Harrelson impression you're ever likely to hear."

"OK," I said, still a bit hesitant, "what's your interest in this?"

"Well," he said, "out here in California we've been trying to find alternative paper sources so we can stop cutting down the old-growth forests and it looks like hemp just might be the answer."

I told him that we were looking at hemp from the Kentucky farmer's perspective, as a possible cash crop alternative to tobacco, but I agreed that hemp had real possibilities as an alternative to wood-based paper.

"Great," he said. "What if I flew out there in a couple of days so we can talk about it?"

I said that that would be fine and that was the end of the conversation. I still didn't really believe it was him. But, sure enough, a few days later, Woody showed up at my house, with his wife Laura and new baby Zoe in tow.

It was strange, but right from the first time we laid eyes on each other, Woody and I made a real connection. It was like he was a brother of mine I hadn't seen in years. He stayed in Lexington for three days and I basically took him through the whole journey of discovery about hemp that I had been through, showing him all the documents I had collected and the equipment and videos we had. By the time I had taught him everything I had learned about industrial hemp, he was as fired up about it as I was.

"I'm convinced this is the answer," he said. "What can I do to help move this along?"

I had been planning to host a conference on industrial hemp in Lexington for some time, so I asked him if he would be a keynote speaker.

"No problem," he said. "Just let me know when you want me."

So Woody went back to L.A. and I got to work on the conference. Well I tell you, with Woody as the star attraction, I didn't have much trouble getting people to attend. Before I knew it, I had farmers, activists, and scientists coming from across the United States and from as far away as Europe and Australia.

As the conference began to really take shape, the words of that one state legislator kept coming back to me, about how we had to get the public educated on the subject before the politicians would do anything about it. So I started racking my brain trying to figure out how best to use Woody's celebrity status to get industrial hemp on the front page of every newspaper in Kentucky, and maybe on a few more besides.

Just before the time for the conference came up, Woody was working on the film *The People vs. Larry Flynt*, so, as you might expect, he was all fired up about the concept of freedom of speech and fighting for your Constitutional rights at that time. We stayed in regular contact by phone and agreed that we needed to do something, a PR stunt or action that involved hemp and some kind of civil disobedience. We didn't want to do anything too extreme, just something interesting enough to get the media out. Then it hit me.

"What about this," I said to Woody. "What if we get some industrial hemp seeds from France, with the doc-

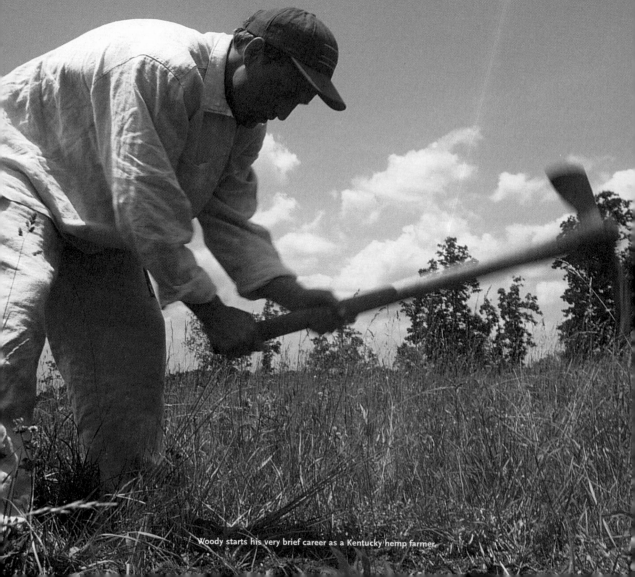

Woody starts his very brief career as a Kentucky hemp farmer.

umentation and everything else to prove they're for industrial use only, then do a press conference with CNN and plant the seeds?"

"Sounds good," Woody said. "What happens after that?"

"Well, since it's illegal to plant hemp for industrial use in Kentucky, I guess the cops'll have to come and arrest you," I answered, half expecting him veto the idea. In his Larry Flynt mindset though, he was up for just about anything. "Cool," he said, "let's do it."

The week of the conference finally came, and Woody and all the speakers and delegates started arriving in town. We kicked the whole thing off on the Thursday with a trip to a middle school in Shelbyville, Kentucky, at one time the center of a thriving hemp industry in that part of the state. The speakers from the conference, including Woody, got up and spoke to the seventh graders about industrial hemp and issues like environmentalism. Having Woody around paid off right away; the kids got a big kick out of having him there, plus we made most front pages across the state the next day. From then on, the eyes of the state media were focused on the International Hemp Conference. Meanwhile, I got on the phone with a friend at CNN to let her know that Woody was going to do "something" during the conference, and that they should all be ready for it.

My little tease worked like a charm; by Saturday morning there were TV news trucks from all over the state and from the major networks parked outside the conference site. On Saturday afternoon, with attorneys in tow and the media in hot pursuit, we headed off to a small town in southeastern Kentucky called Beattyville. Unbeknownst to anyone but a few insiders, Woody had purchased an acre of land there, and that's where we were headed.

We eventually pulled up on the side of this country road and we all got out and walked out into the middle of an unplowed field. Once the TV crews got set up and we were sure that all the reporters had made it, we handed out a news release explaining what Woody was about to do and why he was doing it. Then, with all the cameras rolling, Woody took out a big gardening hoe and started digging in the earth. Once he had the holes dug, he reached in his pocket and pulled out the hemp seeds. The attorney we had with us told him he could only plant four seeds because planting five or more would make it a felony, and that was just more trouble than any of us wanted to get into.

While Woody was preparing to plant the hemp seeds, I took out my cell phone and called the local police to let them know a crime was being committed in a farmer's field just outside of Beattyville—although I think I neglected to mention a movie star was committing the crime and that a small army of reporters was watching him do it. After just a few minutes the county sheriff showed up and walked over to Woody, surveying the situation cautiously. He asked Woody what he was doing and Woody said he was planting industrial hemp seeds. The sheriff wanted to see them and just as quick as he showed them to him, Woody was bent over planting those four seeds. The sheriff then said, "Do you realize you're under arrest?" Woody just politely said, "Yes sir!" With that, the sheriff put the cuffs on Woody, put him in the back of the squad car, and ran him into town to get booked.

We bailed Woody out right away, of course, and that's how our publicity hunt ended, or so we thought. We found out later that planting those seeds was just the beginning of what would turn out to be a long court battle.

From a PR standpoint, the hemp industry couldn't have had a better few days. On Friday we made the front pages for our visit to the school; on Saturday we made them again because people wanted to know what the conference was all about; then we made them once more on Sunday after Woody got arrested. It all went exactly as we'd planned; in just a few days we had the whole state of Kentucky, and lots of other people, talking about industrial hemp. And thanks to Woody putting his freedom on the line to get the word out, we could now say with confidence that most people in the state knew the difference between industrial hemp and marijuana.

After it was all over, Woody went back to California and we went back to our fight to get industrial hemp legalized for cultivation in Kentucky. But things had definitely changed. Because of all the publicity we'd received during the conference, we found that more people knew about the Kentucky Hemp Growers Co-

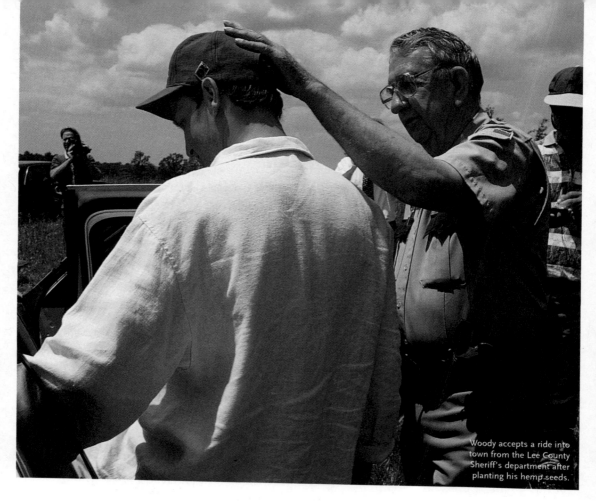

Woody accepts a ride into town from the Lee County Sheriff's department after planting his hemp seeds.

operative and they were much more knowledgeable about the issues surrounding industrial hemp. We also found that more state legislators were willing to talk to us, and we eventually managed to get enough support in the state legislature for a bill allowing the University of Kentucky to undertake a study of the economic viability of industrial hemp. It was still an uphill battle though; the anti-hemp forces fought us every step of the way, using every legislative trick in the book to block or delay anything we put forward.

But Woody's little seed-planting event had taught us a lot about the power of publicity, and we used that knowledge to full advantage. Our next PR challenge was to get four former governors of Kentucky together for a press conference in support of the hemp research legislation, and that's something we never could have done,

or probably would have thought of, before the seed-planting incident.

Later on, when I read in the paper about the DEA going in and destroying a crop of wild hemp on a Native American reserve in North Dakota, we came up with another great idea to get publicity. The way we saw it, Native Americans had been using hemp to make all kinds of things for centuries before the white man ever set foot in North America, so we really didn't have any right to go on their land and cut down their crop. So the Kentucky Hemp Growers Co-operative decided it would replace what the DEA destroyed. We filled a truck with industrial hemp from Canada and drove it from the steps of the Kentucky state house all the way up to North Dakota where we had former Kentucky governor Louie B. Nunn present our replacement hemp to Joe

American Horse and the leadership of the Lakota Nation, right in front of Mount Rushmore. A bit over-the-top, I admit, but we did make the front pages that time too.

Woody's court case, meanwhile, continued to wind its way through the system. He was acquitted in district court because the judge agreed with our argument that the statute didn't mention hemp specifically so Woody didn't break any laws. That ruling was again upheld during our visit to circuit court. After that, the case went to the court of appeal and they basically punted it, I think because they didn't want to have anything to do with a high-profile trial about hemp. The next stop was the Kentucky Supreme Court, and on the very day our hemp legislation was brought up for debate by the state senate, the state Supreme Court ruled that Woody would have to stand trial. We hadn't had so much publicity since Woody actually planted the seeds.

About six months later, almost four years after the actual alleged "crime," we all found ourselves at the Lee County courthouse for Woody's trial. Well, you can imagine they don't get a lot of celebrity trials in Lee County, Kentucky, and that turned this one into an absolute circus, with literally hundreds of people coming from miles around to get a glimpse of the "accused."

The trial itself was one of the best pieces of theatre I've ever witnessed. The sheriff who arrested Woody testified. I testified. Then came the moment everyone was waiting for: Woody took the stand. It was something to see, I'll tell you, Woody getting grilled by this young county prosecutor, who was obviously well aware he was probably trying the most high-profile case of his career. Then, to top it all off, as our lawyer we had the seventy-five-year-old, six-foot-three and 200-plus pound former governor Nunn, one of the most famous governors in the history of Kentucky.

Now that young prosecutor did his level best, but up against Woody, the truth, and Governor Nunn, I don't think he had much of a chance. Naturally, the prosecutor took the line that the opponents of industrial hemp always take: he argued that the whole issue of legalizing industrial hemp for the sake of the farmers was just a ruse; our real goal, he said, was to legalize marijuana.

But when the time came for Governor Nunn to give his closing argument, he made it clear right from the start that he wasn't going to let the "Just Say No" crowd distort the facts.

He started out by giving the court a lesson in civics, explaining to the jury how laws are crafted, debated, and altered by legislators before they are enacted, then enforced by the judiciary. "But when it comes right down to it," he said, resting his hands on the rail and looking right at the jury, "you people get to decide what's right and what's wrong. You people are the last bastion of freedom in this country."

"Your honor," Governor Nunn said, as he walked casually over to the prosecutor's desk. "I've met Mr. Harrelson and I believe he is a fine, upstanding young man. And I don't believe he came to Kentucky to legalize marijuana...

"If I did," he said, raising his voice suddenly and slamming his hand down on the prosecutor's desk, "I'd be sitting at this desk today."

The sound of Governor Nunn hitting the desk made the young prosecutor jump off his chair and it grabbed the attention of everybody in the courtroom. It was incredible to watch, a seventy-five-year-old southern gentleman holding the crowd in the palm of his hand. "Mr. Harrelson shouldn't be convicted of a crime he had no intention of committing," he went on. "He never meant to plant marijuana, and indeed did not plant marijuana, but industrial hemp."

Next, he walked over to the jury and said, "I'd like the members of the jury to take a look at my tie." He held his tie out for the people in the front row to touch and, as the jury members leaned forward to examine it, he explained that the tie was made of hemp fibers and was a gift from Woody.

Finally, he reached in his pocket and pulled out the hemp seed candy bar I'd given him earlier. He opened the wrapper and, holding it up for everyone to see, said, "With the permission of the court"—as if he needed it—"I'm going to take a bite of this hemp bar," which he proceeded to do.

With that, he turned to the jury and said, "Well, ladies and gentlemen of the jury, I've got industrial hemp on me, and now I've got it in me, and I'm sure I've eaten more than four seeds. So, if you lock that man up right there," he said, pointing to Woody, "then you should lock me up too."

Well, after that you could just about hear a pin drop in that courtroom.

After the governor sat down, the judge sent the jury out to deliberate. Woody was pretty cool about it all, but I have to admit, I was on pins and needles as the jury filed out. If they voted to convict, I knew Woody was looking at some jail time and possibly a hefty fine. The jury deliberated for twenty minutes at most, and they surprised everyone when they came back to the court-room so quickly. The jury members just sat stone-faced as the foreman handed the verdict to the judge.

He looked down at the piece of paper and said, "The jury finds the defendant—not guilty."

Well, as soon as the words were out of the judge's mouth the whole courtroom went crazy. People were cheering and clapping as the judge's futile attempt to quiet the courtroom failed. It didn't matter what any-body thought—we won, and the hemp industry was again making headline news.

To tell you the truth, Woody and I had discussed what we wanted the headlines to be months before the trial began. Since the trial was set for July 3, we decided "Independence Day for Kentucky farmers" would be a great headline for the Fourth of July. So when Woody walked out of the courthouse, all the TV and newspaper reporters were waiting for him. Woody walked right up to them with a big smile, leaned into the microphones, and said, "Ladies and gentlemen, today is Independence Day for Kentucky farmers!" That was the sound bite on the evening news and the headline in Kentucky papers the next day. It was amazing to see the headlines come out exactly as we had planned months earlier.

The trial and the publicity it generated pushed the indus-trial hemp movement in Kentucky over the top. Shortly after the trial, the University of Kentucky conducted a sur-vey around the state to find out how people felt about the industrial hemp issue and the results blew us away. The survey found that seventy-seven per cent of Kentuckians either "strongly favored" or "somewhat favored" legislation that would allow farmers to grow industrial hemp. Once we

saw that, we knew we had the ammunition we needed to get the reluctant state legislators onboard.

So we got our hemp legislation introduced again and, with a little arm-twisting by former governor Nunn, it was passed and signed into law by Governor Paul Patton. Most of the legislators voted for the bill because it only authorized hemp "research," and who wants to vote against research? We knew we'd never get a bill passed legalizing hemp production in Kentucky and even if we did, the federal law still prohibited it. So what we did was tack a few lines on the end of the legislation that said, "Kentucky will immediately adopt any and all change in federal hemp legislation," meaning if the feds ever approve hemp farming, Kentucky farmers will be ready to go without further legislative efforts. It wasn't a total victory, but it was a victory nonetheless. And it was sure a hell of a long way from an outright ban, which is what we had when the whole thing started with that newspaper clipping almost ten years before.

• • •

Today, I guess you could say I've evolved into an activist focused on the environment we'll be leaving our chil-dren. But I'm still involved with the hemp industries across North America.

At the moment we're fighting in federal court to stop the DEA from continuing to defame and destroy the U.S. hemp food market. The whole thing is a perfect example of the paranoia that law enforcement agencies foster when it comes to hemp; hemp oil salad dressing is no more dangerous to the nation than poppy seed bagels, but that doesn't stop the DEA from picking on the health food grocery stores selling hemp foods.

Woody and I are also working together with our Lakota friends in a federal lawsuit against the DEA over their illegal destruction of a hemp crop in sovereign ground on the Lakota Reservation. We're hoping to keep the U.S. border open to hemp products from Canada.

But sometimes you just have to wonder why the country known as the "Home of the Brave and Land of the Free" is the only country in the G-8 that doesn't allow its farmers to grow industrial hemp, as if we know something that every other developed nation in the world doesn't know. For me, the fight to legalize

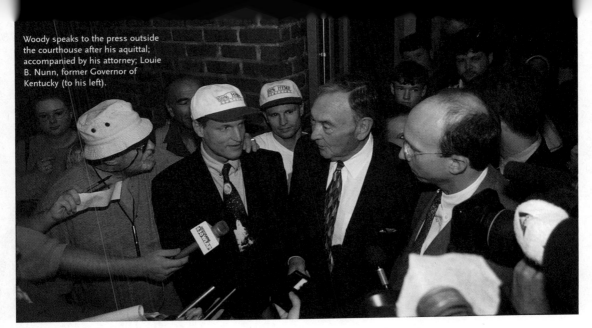

Woody speaks to the press outside the courthouse after his aquittal; accompanied by his attorney; Louie B. Nunn, former Governor of Kentucky (to his left).

industrial hemp in the United States is really about freedom itself. As an American, it bothers me that our farmers can't grow a plant that farmers in Third World communist countries have been growing for years. Does that sound like a free country?

Any way you look at it, the government's position on hemp is simply not rational, and I believe it's worth fighting to change that position. I also believe it should alarm every American that there are politicians and government agencies hell-bent on maintaining the status quo, even when the status quo makes no sense.

Saying industrial hemp and marijuana are the same thing over and over again doesn't make it so: THC is the element in marijuana that makes you stoned, but industrial hemp only contains about one per cent THC, while marijuana can contain more than twenty per cent. Meanwhile we're missing out on a benign plant that has innumerable practical uses and can be grown with minimal impact on the environment.

In light of these facts, I don't know why some people fight so hard against industrial hemp—maybe it's because they're fighting for their jobs and fighting to preserve their budgets; maybe it's because they're under pressure from industries that feel threatened by hemp; or maybe it's because they just don't want to admit that they're wrong.

In the meantime, I'm just going to continue the job I started in Kentucky so many years ago: telling the truth,

educating people, raising awareness.

That has led me to what I'm doing now, helping to develop new, environmentally friendly technologies that will reduce our impact on the planet. One of the most important things I learned during the hemp fight in Kentucky was the power of creating positive alternatives to our old, polluting industries. That's what drew me to the hemp issue in the first place—the idea that it could help farmers and the environment at the same time. The new projects I'm working on will do the same thing, creating real examples of sustainability that will provide cleaner air and water for everyone.

I think my experiences also taught me the power of a few people to make a difference, if you just put your mind to it. Somebody has got to speak up and say the emperor's got no clothes, and I guess I can do that as well as anybody else. All of us can. Woody feels the same way, and that's probably why we made such a strong connection when we stood up together for what we believed in in that field in Kentucky.

He was there for me, so I was only too happy to stand up with him on the SOL Tour, and I'm sure we'll be fighting the good fight together for years to come.

Joe Hickey is a Board member of the Ruckus Society and Executive Director of the Kentucky Hemp Growers Co-operative Association

207

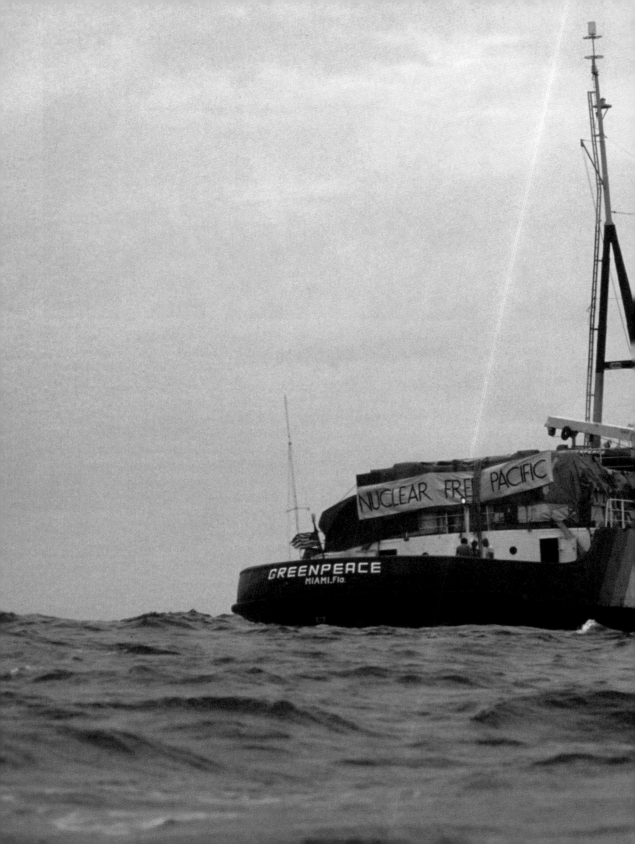

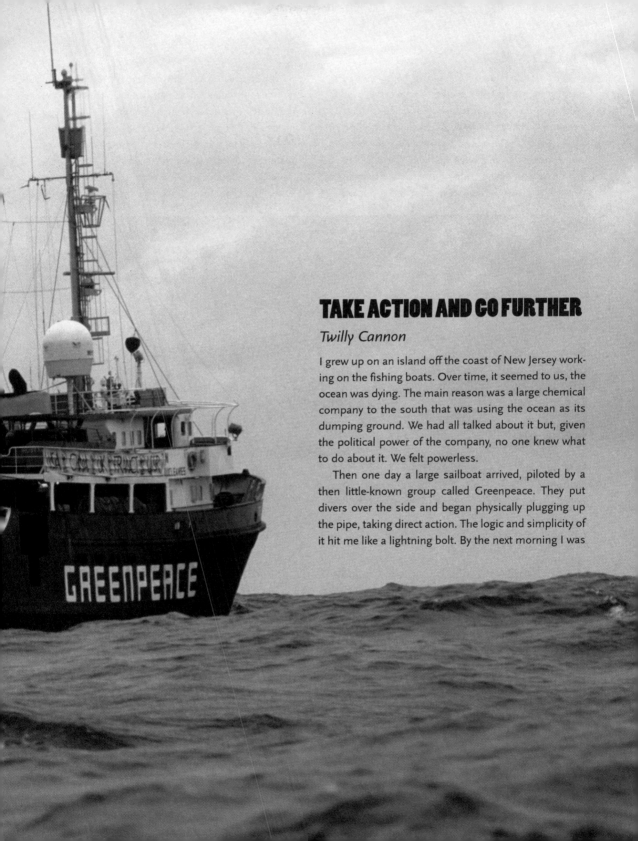

TAKE ACTION AND GO FURTHER

Twilly Cannon

I grew up on an island off the coast of New Jersey working on the fishing boats. Over time, it seemed to us, the ocean was dying. The main reason was a large chemical company to the south that was using the ocean as its dumping ground. We had all talked about it but, given the political power of the company, no one knew what to do about it. We felt powerless.

Then one day a large sailboat arrived, piloted by a then little-known group called Greenpeace. They put divers over the side and began physically plugging up the pipe, taking direct action. The logic and simplicity of it hit me like a lightning bolt. By the next morning I was onboard doing whatever I could to help—and by that evening I was in jail with the rest of the crew.

My cellmates all seemed pretty psyched-up, but I was feeling low. Had we really accomplished anything? After all, we were in jail and the company was removing our plug. Soon after our release, I realized why my new friends were so elated: it didn't matter that the plug had come out because what had also come out was *the idea*

power of direct action. In those years, standing on the shoulders of giants, I've seen action play a critical role in stopping nuclear testing, ending the dumping of wastes in the oceans, greatly reducing whaling, banning the most dangerous common chemicals, and in other instances too numerous to recount.

History abounds with examples of action changing the world. The fights against slavery, colonialism, and war, and

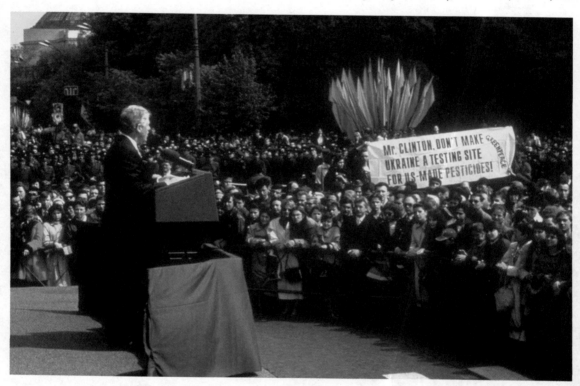

that the pipe could be shut down. Once they saw that something could be done, people started actually talking about a day when the ocean would no longer be used as a chemical toilet. Inspired by the courage of the Greenpeace activists, others began to take action. It took a couple more years of determined fighting, but that pipe was eventually and permanently shut down.

I went on to work with Greenpeace for over twenty years, and time and again I've seen the transformative

for civil rights were all marked by the extensive use of direct action. What puzzles me is, in spite of all these examples, you still hear people saying, "What's the use? Protesting will never change anything." Imagine what our world would look like if Gandhi or Martin Luther King had felt that way.

One of the reasons for this pessimism, I believe, is how we are raised to view struggle. We are raised on the myth of what I call "the single-combat warrior"—St. George versus the dragon; David versus Goliath; the two gunfighters squaring off in the street. The contest is short, the results clear and decisive.

In the real world, the fights worth fighting are rarely short and decisive. Many take years of struggle. For example, I was privileged to be in on the endgame of the campaign against nuclear testing—sailing into the French nuclear test site in the Pacific, trying to prevent the bomb going off. Each morning the protest fleet would gather to plan the day's actions. I remember standing on deck, watching the dozens of different vessels rendezvous, and thinking, "This may be the last time this fleet may have to gather." By the time the campaign was over, the momentum towards a comprehensive test ban was unstoppable.

Pretty heady stuff. But what's important to remember is—as I said above—I was standing on the shoulders of giants. For over thirty years prior, other activists had fought the fight I was now a part of. Likewise, I was in on the end of the campaign to stop the dumping of nuclear waste in the ocean—the close of another thirty-year campaign.

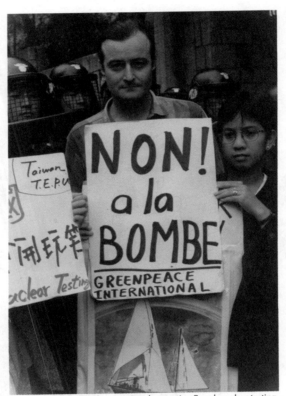
Twilly at the French embassy in Seoul protesting French nuclear testing.

There are times when it's very fulfilling to be an activist; I was very lucky to be in on the gratifying ends of these great campaigns. But in most cases, one has to find sustenance outside of the prospect of quick victory. One has to, as Camus put it, "struggle without hope." I know that sounds pretty bleak, but even without victory there is a reward.

My work with Greenpeace has taken me all over the world. I've been able to experience many different peoples and cultures. (I've been able to experience a lot of different jail cells, too.) Throughout the years I've been fortunate to work with some incredible activists. We've struggled, suffered, feared, and grown together. We're a community.

This is the reward I was talking about. The experience of struggle, alone and together, not only made me who I am today, but also allowed me to grow into, and with, this magical community. Activism gave me the opportunity to experience things I never would have if I had stayed on the sidelines. It has allowed me—a kid from a small fishing village—to see places I likely never would have otherwise. And, once in a while, I was lucky enough to witness a victory.

So whenever I hear anyone say, "What's the use?" I tell them this: forget the hackneyed pessimism that says you can't make a difference; that's just what the bad guys want you to think. Find your passion, dream your dream—and then take action. You can change the world. The famous writer Goethe had it exactly right when he said, "Whatever you think you can do or believe you can do, begin it. Action has magic, grace and power in it."

Howard "Twilly" Cannon is a co-founder of the Ruckus Society and former skipper of the Greenpeace vessel Rainbow Warrior.

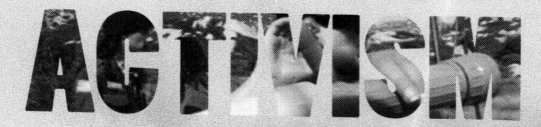ACTIVISM

It was really significant for me that we started our little bike trip down the West Coast in the great city of Seattle. The SOL Tour was really about encouraging people to stand up and take personal responsibility for saving our planet, and after what happened at the World Trade Organization (WTO) Summit in Seattle in November 1999, that city has become a big symbol of that kind of responsibility. In fact, when it comes to people standing up for what's right, just the name Seattle carries as much meaning for today's generation of activists as names like Selma and Kent State do for the children of the 1960s.

For me, what happened in Seattle during the WTO Summit was like the first big, shining neon sign at the dawn of the twenty-first century that the youth of today (and the young at heart) have what it takes to say to the power brokers of the world, "We've had enough and we're not putting up with your shit anymore."

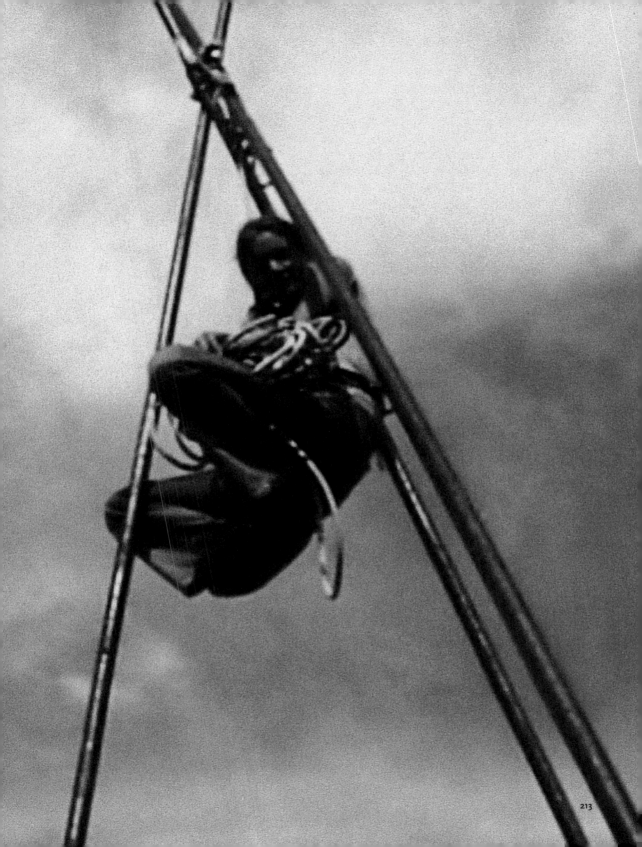

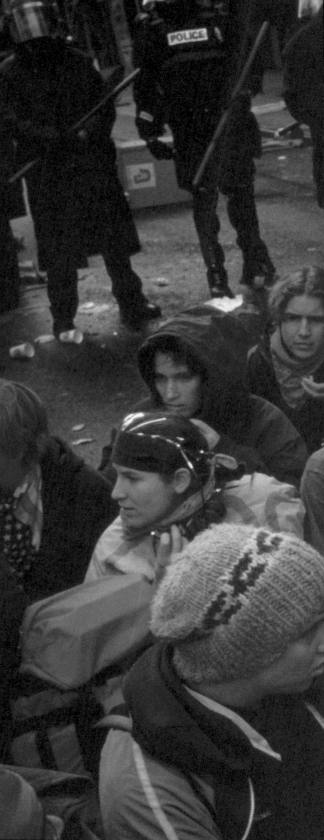

I wasn't in Seattle for the WTO Summit, and I regret that because I think—I hope—that it marked a new beginning for social activism in the United States and around the world. I did follow it all on TV and the Internet though, and it did my heart good to see that there are people in the world, lots of them, who are aware of the terrible effect unchecked industrial activity is having on our environment, who realize how multinational corporations exploit workers in poor countries just to boost their bottom line, and who understand that it's our own elected officials who help make it all happen. It made me feel even better when those same people managed to shut the whole circus down through sheer force of will.

Like I say, I wasn't in Seattle for the WTO, but my good friend and fellow SOL Tour companion Joe Hickey, who I call the father of the hemp movement, was there, and we spent a lot of time talking about it during those long hours cycling down the coast. It must've been an amazing experience for him, because it's an amazing story to hear. He told me about how he ran through the streets of the city with groups of young people protesting, setting up roadblocks, trying to block the entrances to the buildings where the Summit was being held, and trying to connect with the foreign delegates to convince them to join the protests.

"It was fun," Joe told me, "but it was more than fun."

It was inspiring too, he said, because you really got the sense among the people out in the streets that they understood the issues and they really wanted to make a difference. "They cared," Joe said. "Even when the cops were beatin' on them, they wouldn't leave because they cared."

Like most people, I only saw the events in Seattle through the corporate media filter, so I didn't know what really went on there. But Joe told me it was a lot worse than it looked on the six o'clock news, and I thought that looked pretty bad. The thing about Seattle was, the protesters were really organized, and they were moving around in coordinated groups, each with a specific assignment to disrupt the Summit, and the groups kept in touch with each other by cell phone. That made it really hard for the cops to stay on top of the protest-

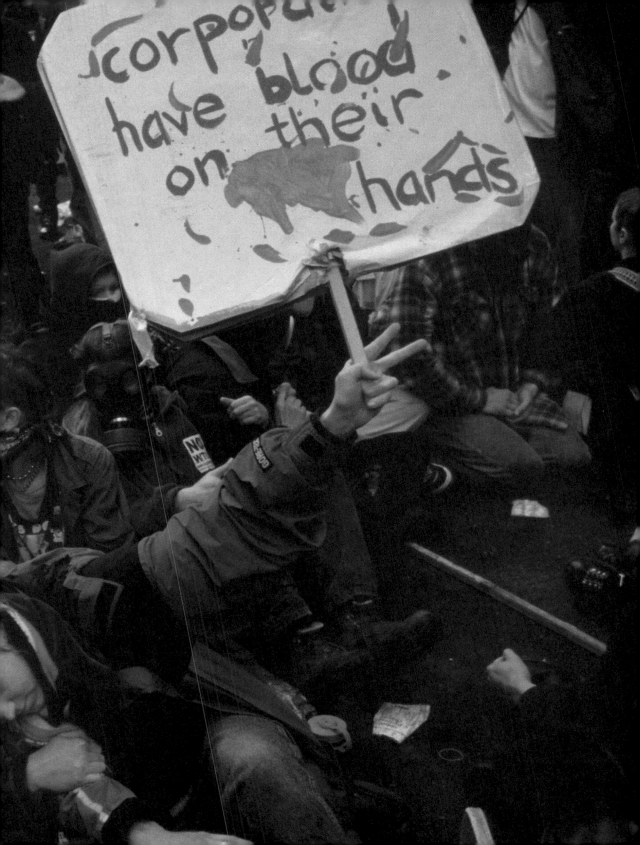

ers and keep everything under control. And when the cops started to realize they were up against some serious opposition, they just went crazy.

Joe said the cops started out trying to move the protesters physically, but as soon as they got one group of protesters away from the Summit site, another group would move right in behind them. That's when the batons came out. But when that didn't do the trick either, the cops decided to use tear gas and rubber bullets to establish a kind of buffer zone between the protesters and the key Summit buildings. Then the chief of police called a curfew and everybody had to be off the streets by 9:00 at night. Joe told me about how he watched the cops clear the streets: They'd line up across the road from one side to the other—a phalanx, I think they call it—dressed in these black Darth Vader masks and body armor, then just walk up the street smacking their batons against their riot shields. Anybody who was stupid enough to get in their way just got clubbed down and walked over.

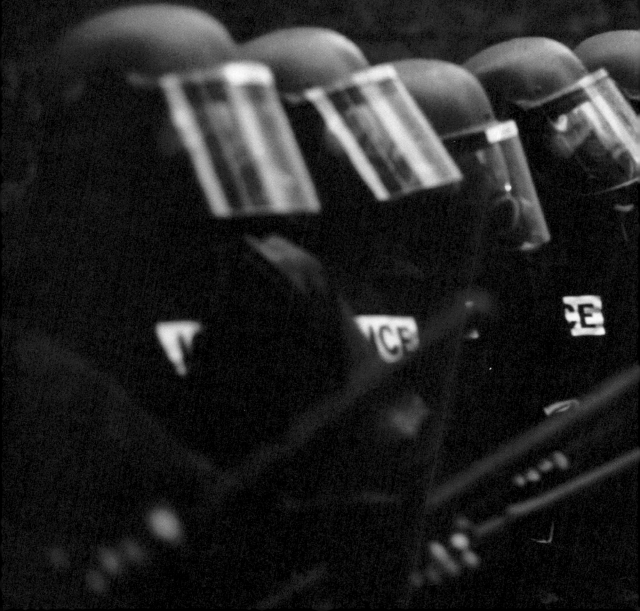

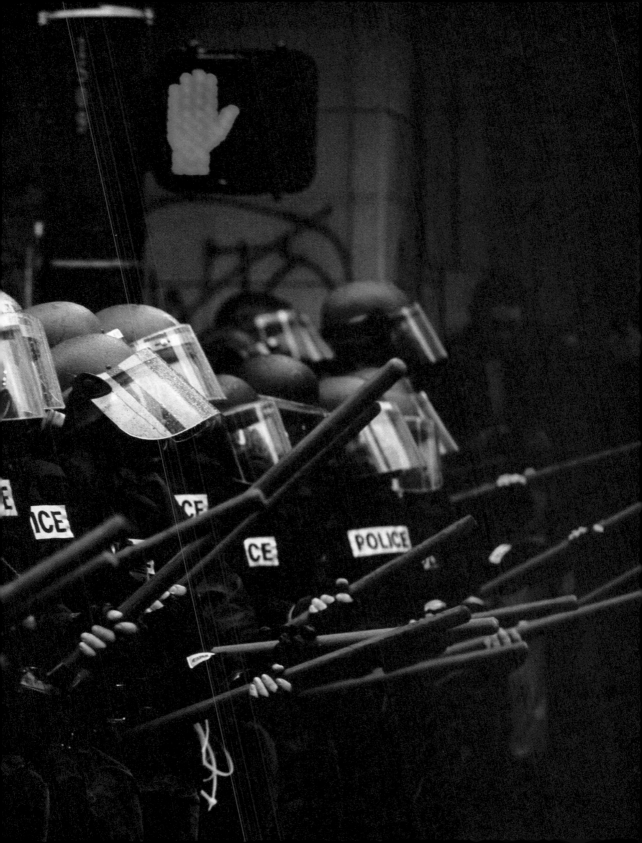

"I had to keep telling myself I was in the United States," Joe told me, "and not in Guatemala or Argentina or some Third World dictatorship like that."

At one point, he said, when the cops were driving the protesters down the side streets, some of the local people who actually lived there came out of their houses and apartments and tried to get between the cops and the protesters. He said the citizens of Seattle were actually yelling at their own cops: "We pay your wages, and you're not going to turn our neighborhood into a police state."

Joe told me about how he and a bunch of other protesters got caught down a side street by the cops, so they just sat down in the road with some of the local citizens who came out to try to protect them and started a kind of standoff with the police. They were there for a few hours and a couple of Seattle city council members even came down to join them. At one point, he said, one of the protesters suggested that they all try to diffuse the tension with a little love, so they all started singing Christmas carols. That must have been quite a scene—all these young protesters sitting in the middle of road with little old ladies and parents with kids from the area singing *Silent Night*, while just a few yards away there's this line of cops with clubs and riot gear just waiting for the order to move in.

They got their wish eventually. Joe said a cop on a bullhorn announced that they had five minutes to clear the street—then four, three, two, one. The cops started to beat their shields with their clubs, but the people just kept singing. Suddenly the guy on the horn yelled, "Clear!" and the goons moved in. The tear gas started flying and the batons started swinging, and for about ten minutes, Joe said, that street in Seattle looked like a war zone.

When it was all over, the street was clear all right, but that was the final straw for the local citizens. Lots of people got hurt in that standoff with the cops, and lots of them weren't even protesters. In fact, one of the city councilors who joined the sit-in got hit in the back with a tear gas canister. After that episode, the people of Seattle finally spoke up and

said, "Enough. No more tear gas. No more batons. We don't want this shit in our city."

When the cops realized the citizens wouldn't stand for the strong-arm tactics anymore, they told the WTO they couldn't guarantee security, and that was it. They had to shut it down, and it was all because the people, just everyday people, cared enough to get involved. I tip my hat to everyone who was a part of what happened during the WTO Summit in Seattle, and I believe that's just the kind of involvement we're going to need from everybody in this country if we're going to take our planet back from the Beast.

I guess I've developed a bit of a reputation over the years for being a social activist, and I am proud of the small contributions I've been able to make. But I wasn't always out there fighting the good fight. For most of my life, I was like most people, just doing what I needed to do to make a living and living my life in the cocoon I created for myself. I always had strong opinions about things—politics, the environment—but never so strong that I wanted to put myself out there in front like some kind of activist poster boy. Besides, I thought, who the hell is going to listen to some crazy actor anyway. That all changed during the Persian Gulf War back in 1991; that's when I got sucked into a situation that really made me realize I did have a voice and that it was up to me whether I was going to use it to make a difference in the world or not.

The Persian Gulf War bothered me for a lot of reasons. I mean, I knew Saddam Hussein was a bad guy and that the world couldn't stand by while he invaded Kuwait, but the whole thing just seemed so convenient to me. After all, it was the CIA that brought Hussein and the Baath Party to power. It is their M.O.—bring in a brutal dictator to maintain order while the resources are taken by the Beast. If Kuwait and Iraq weren't sitting on most of the world's oil reserves, we probably wouldn't have given a shit what Hussein did. Sure, we like to act like the great liberator and defender of human rights, but in the end, it was a war about oil, and

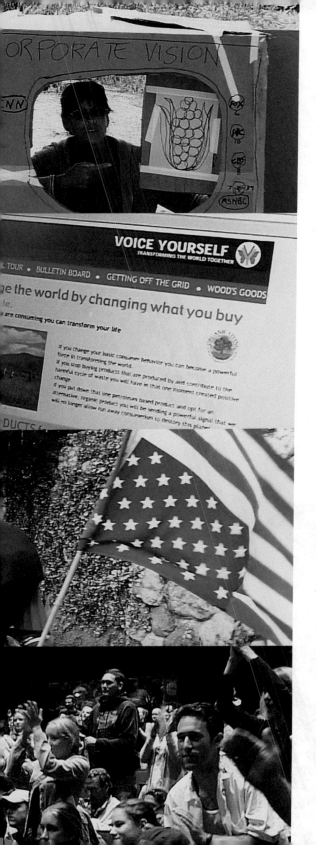

that bothered me. On top of that, it gave our military-industrial complex a chance to gain billions more in funding as well as a perfect excuse to go in there and try out their new toys on some real targets, and that bothered me too.

I remember the war had just started and I got a call from a friend of mine, Clem Frank, who told me that there was a bunch of students doing an anti-war sit-in over at UCLA and he asked me if I wanted to go and check it out. I don't know why but I went over there with him and the next thing I knew the place was crawling with TV cameras because "Woody from *Cheers* is leading a protest at UCLA." Then a couple of pro-war people showed up and pretty soon I was shooting my mouth off, as I'm wont to do, and the whole thing got way more heated than I ever could've imagined. But that was just the beginning.

The day after the protest, I'm thinking, "OK, that was weird, but it's all over now." Then I get a call from these people in New Orleans who want to withdraw their invitation for me to ride in a special float in the Mardi Gras parade, which I had already committed to doing. Then I get a call from my agent who informs me that the Miller Lite commercial I was going to do, which was going to be my second one, just got pulled by Miller because of my "controversial views." After that the phone was ringing off the hook all day with various people telling me, "Man, you better shut up; you're pissing a lot of people off," and "You could lose your career over this."

I couldn't believe it: in twenty-four hours I went from Woody Harrelson, actor, to Woody Harrelson, dangerous war protester. What pissed me off the most about it all, though, was that I was just saying what I really felt, and now there were all these people trying to silence me. It was pretty obvious that I had a choice to make: I could shut my mouth and keep doing beer commercials—go along to get along—or I could stand up for what I believe in and take my chances.

"You know what," I thought, "I've had a great career [and this was more than ten years ago]. I've had more success than I ever could've anticipated. I'm just going to stick to my guns, and if I lose my career, then I don't need it anyway." (And besides, Miller beer may be the worst ever made.)

That's the way I've looked at it ever since. Somehow I've managed to stay in the acting business, but I've probably done a lot less work than I could have if I'd just been a good soldier all these years instead of an "actor/activist." But looking back now, I wouldn't want it any other way. Sure, it's nice to get lots of work, but that's not my top priority. I mean, I look at it like this: my Mother's being raped. How can I worry about making a beer commercial when my Mother's being raped?

So I've tried to do as much as I could over the years to lend my voice to the chorus, for what it's worth. If people will listen to me because they've seen me on TV or in the movies, then I figure it's my duty to get up there and say the right things. It's the least I can do to help out the people who are on the front lines fighting the good fight, people like Julia Butterfly Hill, who lived in that redwood tree for almost two years to protest clear-cutting, and people like the protesters who braved tear gas and batons to shut down the WTO Summit in Seattle.

I've been lucky enough to hang out with those people on the front lines now and again, and you won't

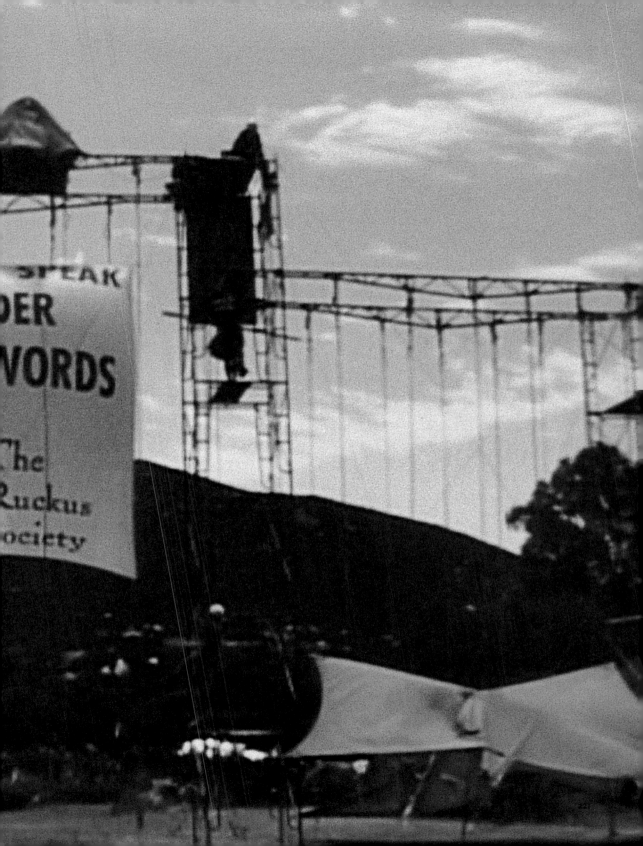

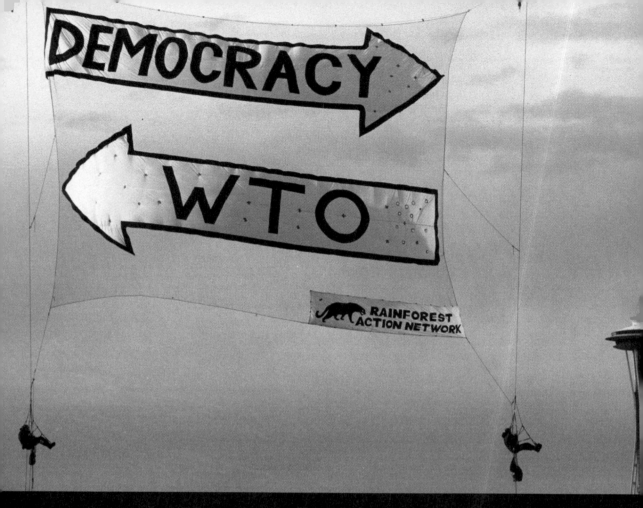

find more dedicated people anywhere on earth. And they know how to have fun, too—that deep down fun that comes after a hard day of fighting for your Mother. In 1996 I climbed the Golden Gate Bridge with some really cool people from groups like Earth First, the Ruckus Society, and Rainforest Action Network to protest logging in California's ancient Headwaters Forest, and it was an amazing experience. We got arrested, of course, but nobody got hurt and I think we really got people thinking about the issue, so it was all worth it for me. Another time I got in some trouble in Kentucky for planting some industrial hemp seeds and I got arrested for that too. But that's how I met Joe Hickey of the Kentucky Hemp Growers' Co-operative and the hemp activist lawyer Tom Ballanco, who became personal friends, so that experience was more than worth the hassle as well.

For me, the rewards for standing up for what I believe is right have far outweighed any material wealth I might have gained if I'd kept my mouth shut.

So when people call me an "activist," I'm particularly proud of that. At least it means I'm trying to be part of the solution. I think most people would agree that the system we have in the world today, the one run by the WTO, the World Bank, the G-8, and the multinational corporations that bankroll those organizations, is fucked up—it's bad for the planet itself and bad for the vast majority of people living on it. But I believe we can turn it around. I believe in the power of transformation.

I'm a non-violent activist because I believe that non-violent protest, even radical non-violent protest like we saw in Seattle, can transform our adversaries, can win them over rather than defeat them. We have to keep

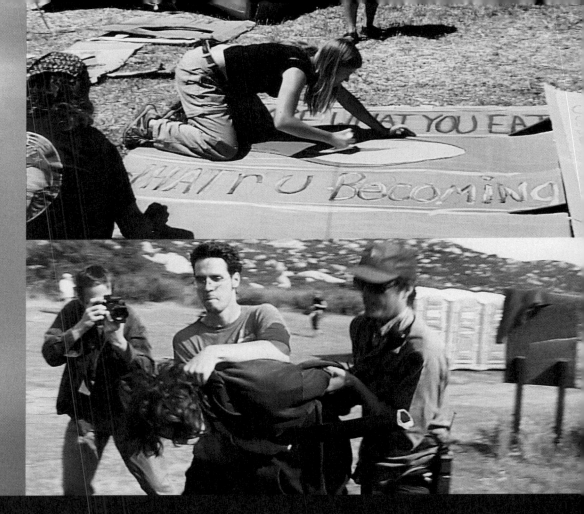

those lines of communication open. I mean, if people are willing to step out of their box, with openness and in the spirit of co-operation, to talk about alternative solutions, then I'm willing to talk to anybody. And you know, I'd much rather win over somebody with the logic of my argument and celebrate that victory together than to just say, "I'm right. You're wrong," and shut them out. That's how the Beast does business, and we know how well that approach works.

That doesn't mean I don't think there are a few bad people on the planet who won't listen to any opinion that contradicts their own, no matter how much sense it makes. Mostly though, I think we just get caught up in bad systems. It's like we get so hooked into doing things the wrong way—like building our whole society around the consumption of fossil fuels—that we don't

know how to get out of it. Then, without thinking, we pass that negative pathology on to the next generation. Well, I believe that we can transform the way people think about things if we continue to challenge those negative systems and offer viable alternatives. That's what they were doing in Seattle: the protesters were asking the WTO delegates to take a good long look at what they were doing in the world and what motivates them; they were asking them to wake up and acknowledge the fact that multinational corporations are destroying our planet and making obscene profits through the misery of poor people. That's the truth. And connecting people to the truth is the essence of activism for me.

You know, it's so easy to put your blinders on and pretend everything is just fine, especially when you've got the people in power telling you over and over that

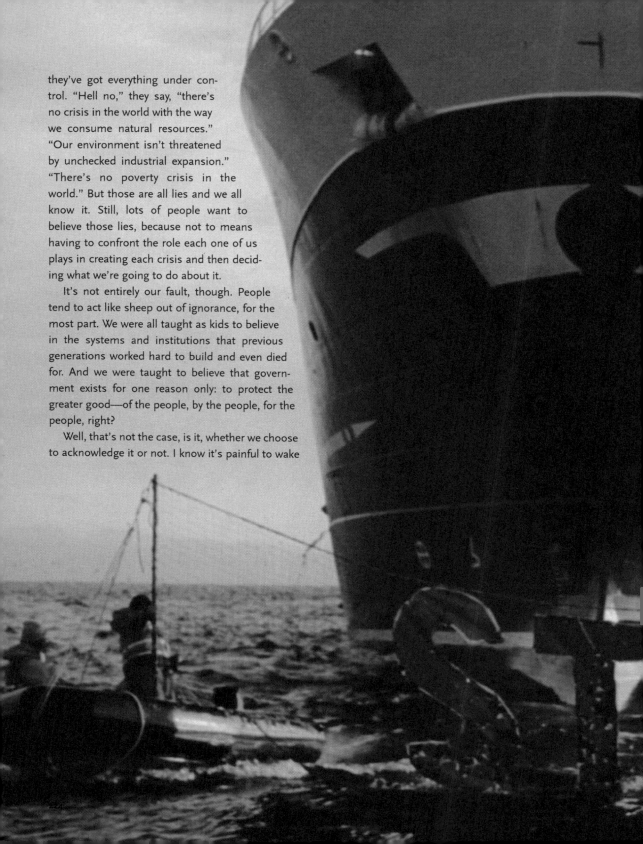

they've got everything under control. "Hell no," they say, "there's no crisis in the world with the way we consume natural resources." "Our environment isn't threatened by unchecked industrial expansion." "There's no poverty crisis in the world." But those are all lies and we all know it. Still, lots of people want to believe those lies, because not to means having to confront the role each one of us plays in creating each crisis and then deciding what we're going to do about it.

It's not entirely our fault, though. People tend to act like sheep out of ignorance, for the most part. We were all taught as kids to believe in the systems and institutions that previous generations worked hard to build and even died for. And we were taught to believe that government exists for one reason only: to protect the greater good—of the people, by the people, for the people, right?

Well, that's not the case, is it, whether we choose to acknowledge it or not. I know it's painful to wake

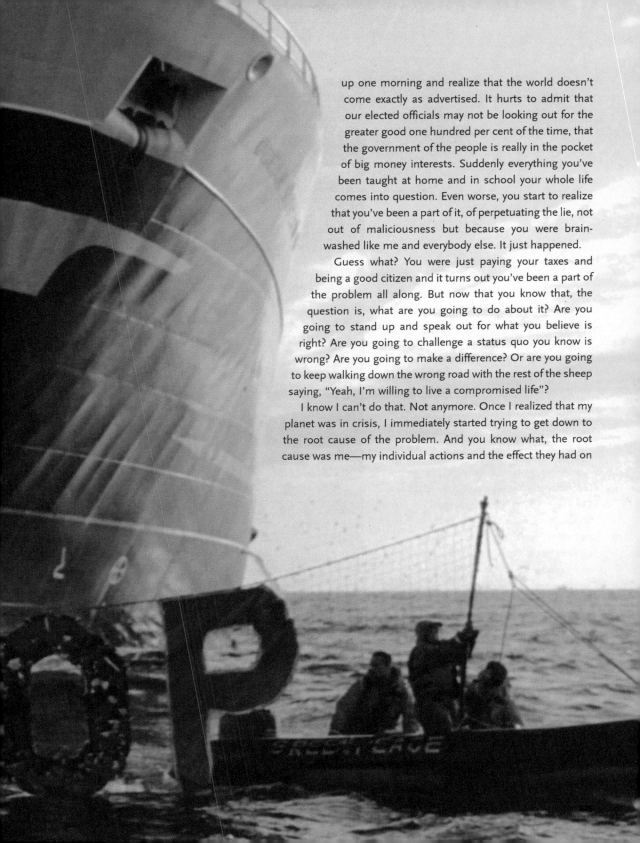

up one morning and realize that the world doesn't come exactly as advertised. It hurts to admit that our elected officials may not be looking out for the greater good one hundred per cent of the time, that the government of the people is really in the pocket of big money interests. Suddenly everything you've been taught at home and in school your whole life comes into question. Even worse, you start to realize that you've been a part of it, of perpetuating the lie, not out of maliciousness but because you were brainwashed like me and everybody else. It just happened.

Guess what? You were just paying your taxes and being a good citizen and it turns out you've been a part of the problem all along. But now that you know that, the question is, what are you going to do about it? Are you going to stand up and speak out for what you believe is right? Are you going to challenge a status quo you know is wrong? Are you going to make a difference? Or are you going to keep walking down the wrong road with the rest of the sheep saying, "Yeah, I'm willing to live a compromised life"?

I know I can't do that. Not anymore. Once I realized that my planet was in crisis, I immediately started trying to get down to the root cause of the problem. And you know what, the root cause was me—my individual actions and the effect they had on the world. On the other hand, I figured out that the solution to the problem was me too, if I decided to be. I guess that's how I hit on the concept of simple organic living: it's just each one of us figuring out what we can do as individuals to effect positive change. We all have a role to play, and I think part of our life's work is to find out what that role is. Shit, that's as grassroots as activism gets.

The bottom line is, the system needs an enema. The way our species is running this planet is screwed from the ground up, and if we're going to wait for change to come from within the system, we might as well start apologizing to our kids and grandkids for the mess right now. No one is going to save the planet for us. There's no talking head on the box who's going to make everything all right. If we want to live in a world that's better than the one we live in right now, it's up to each one of us to create that world.

In the end, that's what's going to change things for the better: action on an individual basis with a collective vision for the future. That's what's going to help us find a balance between ourselves and the natural world. That's what's going to help us change the way we relate to one another and strike some kind of balance with our brothers and sisters throughout the planet.

No one should kid themselves though; being an activist is hard. It takes courage to stand up for what you believe in, especially when that view is not the popular one. It takes courage to speak up, and it takes even more courage to act. Sometimes you have to take risks, and you have to be willing to deal with the repercussions of your words or actions. That might mean being ridiculed or rejected by your family and friends; it might

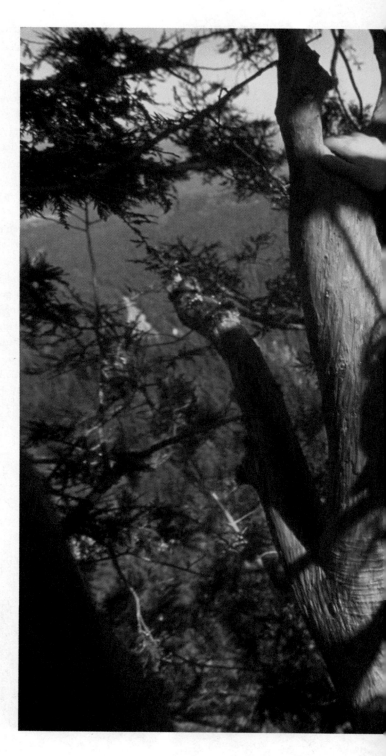

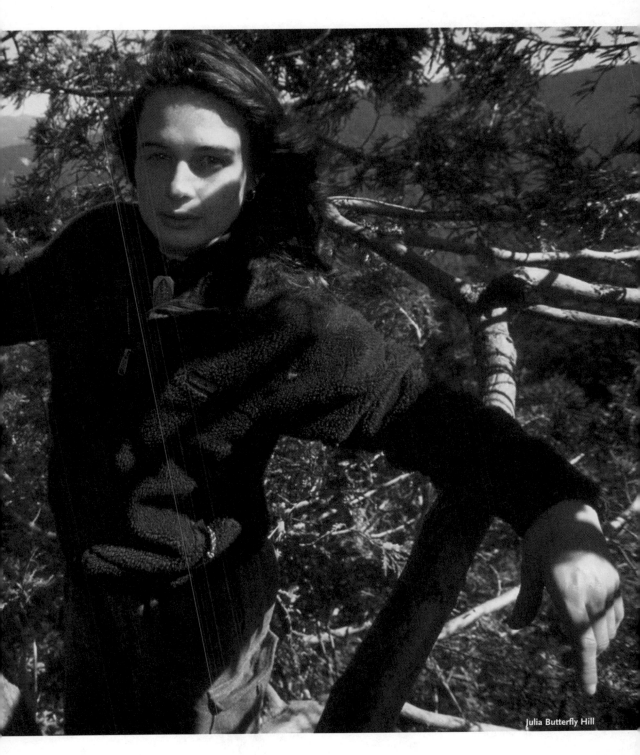

Julia Butterfly Hill

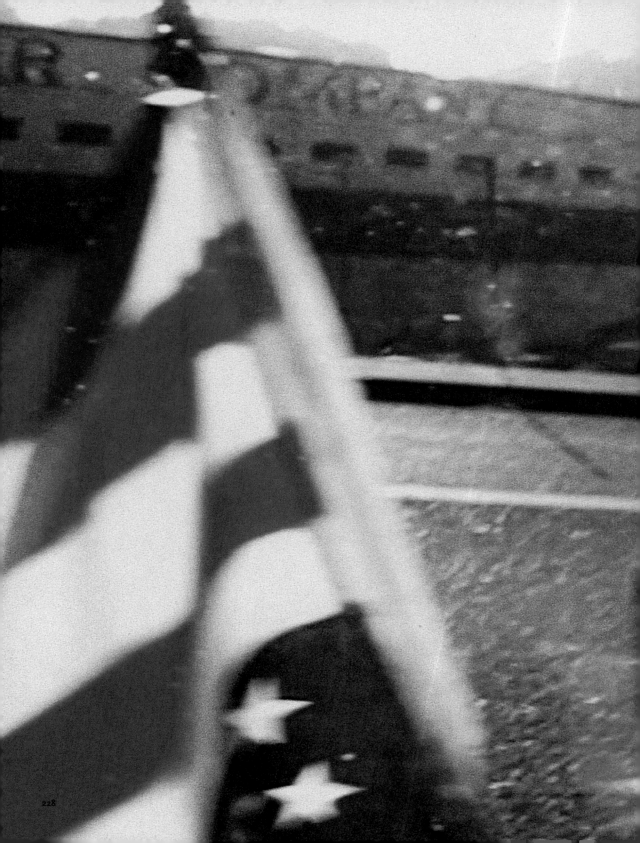

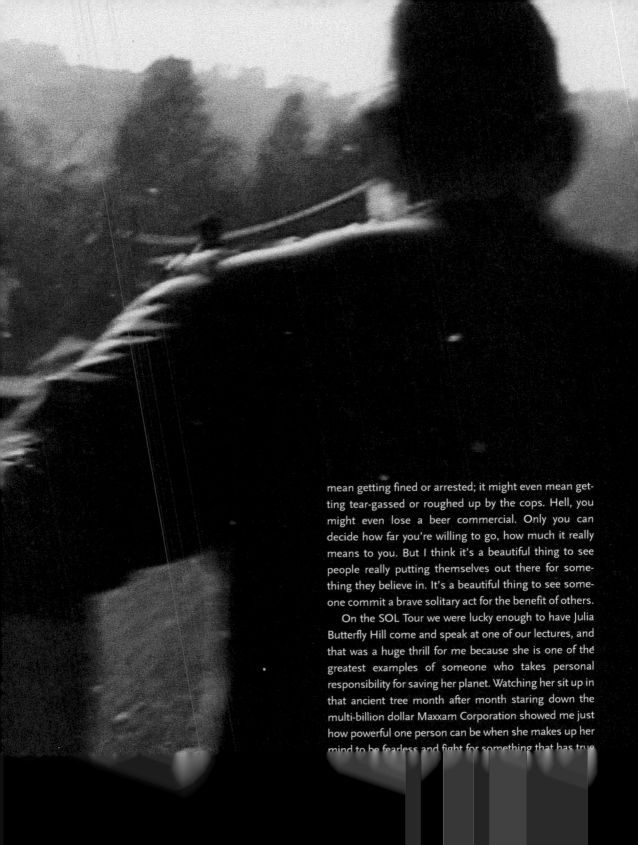

mean getting fined or arrested; it might even mean getting tear-gassed or roughed up by the cops. Hell, you
might even lose a beer commercial. Only you can
decide how far you're willing to go, how much it really
means to you. But I think it's a beautiful thing to see
people really putting themselves out there for something they believe in. It's a beautiful thing to see someone commit a brave solitary act for the benefit of others.

On the SOL Tour we were lucky enough to have Julia
Butterfly Hill come and speak at one of our lectures, and
that was a huge thrill for me because she is one of the
greatest examples of someone who takes personal
responsibility for saving her planet. Watching her sit up in
that ancient tree month after month staring down the
multi-billion dollar Maxxam Corporation showed me just
how powerful one person can be when she makes up her
mind to be fearless and fight for something that has true

In her talk, Julia said something that really cut to the core of what activism is all about. She said that every time we point at things that are wrong in the world, there are three fingers pointing back at us. "You can't just point at the people who are wrong and say, 'Fix it,'" she said. "You must become a part of the solution every moment of every single day. That's your power."

I think it's true that we tend to forget just how much power each individual has to effect change in the world. People like Julia are a living example of the fact that we are all powerful beyond our wildest dreams. We have the power to change the world because everything we do and say and even our inactions make a difference in the way other people act. It's like Julia says: "If you walk away from an injustice, you are a part of it." Why? Because every moment we're on this planet we have a choice to make, and every choice has an impact.

Because we have the freedom to make choices, we also have a responsibility to make good ones. You always hear the George Bushes of the world talk about how America is the greatest country in the world because "we've got the freedom to choose." But you never hear them talk about the responsibility that should go with that freedom, the responsibility to choose carefully, consciously, respectfully, and compassionately. Politicians don't talk about that because most people don't want to hear it. They don't want you to get all heavy with them because it might kill their wild consumer buzz, and the Beast sure wouldn't want that.

I like to stay light and have fun as much as anybody—maybe a little more—but I also understand that we've got to be smart about it too. When you choose to drive around in a massive SUV, it means some little kid in the inner city needs to get an inhaler just so he can run around the playground. Don't believe that? Well, all of us living today are living with the consequences of the bad choices made by the people who came before us. I didn't decide that L.A. would work better if it was designed to let people drive their cars everywhere instead of ride mass transit. But I pay for that decision every time I take a breath on a hot summer afternoon in L.A. And in exactly the same way, those who come after us will have to live with the choices we make today. So what do you think? Should we continue to compound the errors of the past, or should we change direction?

I think the answer to that question is pretty obvious, and I believe social activism, both individual and collective, is going to play a key role in getting this ship turned around. The great thing about it is the alternative solutions that can pull us back from the brink are already out there just waiting for us to take advantage of them. That's why I believe my primary role as an activist is to educate people about those alternatives, to show them there is another way. That's what the SOL Tour was all about: traveling in a bus powered by biodiesel, using photovoltaic panels to make electricity, talking about growing food in partnership with nature, and coming together as a community of like-minded individuals based on equality and trust. It was social activism on wheels.

Unfortunately, I think the incredible alternative solutions that do exist get lost in the noise of protest sometimes. Too often, activists are shown as a kind of negative force that's always saying "Stop," "Turn back," "You're wrong." Part of that is the corporate media's handiwork, but we don't help our own cause a lot of the time. The six o'clock news often just focuses on the "protesters" and ignores the issues that led to the protest. To lots of non-activists, it seems activists are always pointing the finger, like a bunch of hypercritical old curmudgeons who can't agree with anything or cut anybody any slack. I also think oftentimes activists take themselves pretty seriously that way. And when that's all people think of when they think of an activist, what gets lost are the incredible solutions, the extraordinary world vision that we're beginning to bring together based on compassion, sharing, human rights, and ecological sustainability.

We tried to avoid projecting the "liberal hippie freak" thing on the SOL Tour, though that may be an apt name for all of us. We were never shy about being seen as people who have a problem with the narrow corporate paradigm that prevails in the world right now, but it wasn't just about that; it was about the alternatives to that. And I think any time people can work in a positive direction and demonstrate solutions through their actions, that's the kind of activism that transforms people. Don't get me wrong, I wouldn't mind going to jail again under the right circumstances, and sometimes that's what's required to make the point you're trying to make. It's just that, for me, nothing beats being able to show somebody a better way.

While it's true that the rewards of standing up for what you believe in are great, that doesn't mean that being a social activist isn't sometimes a thankless task. I know there are a lot of people who feel totally helpless against the system. I've felt that way myself sometimes, like a lone voice in the wilderness. It's also frustrating to see all these individual activist groups fighting for recognition and the media spotlight. It's like they all have their own constituencies in a way, just like separate political parties. I often think to myself: Man, what if all these social activists could get together and focus that energy like they did in Seattle, but not just for a few days—every day. We'd be a force to be reckoned with, wouldn't we?

Well, the good news is you're not a lone voice in the wilderness, and we know that because there are so many non-profit and activist groups out there fighting the good fight, whether it's for the environment, women's rights, housing, or whatever. Our voices may drown each other out every now and again, but we're all cut from the same cloth, we all have the same basic vision for the future.

I read a great book one time called *State of the World,* and in that book the authors talk about a segment of society they call the "cultural creatives." Cultural creatives are people who are dissatisfied with the current system and the institutions that govern our society. They want to create a new culture that embraces alternative solutions. The book's authors estimate that the cultural creatives actually make up about twenty-six per cent of the population. The most interesting thing about these people, though, is that they have no idea there are so many other people who think like they do. Well, I think it's time we started to hook up.

Actually, that's one of the best things about getting involved in activist causes: it allows you to meet so many like-minded people. I don't know how many people I met on the SOL Tour—thousands easily—who had found some way to get involved in being part of the solution. In fact, I was really amazed to see how many

kids and young people are starting things on their own in junior high or high school or college—starting an ecology club, or a human rights club, or a cycling club, even yoga. And they'll carry those ideas with them throughout their lives.

I know you hear all the time about voter apathy, but I found that people are actually enthusiastic about saving the planet—I guess because they've given up on government. They want to be inspired and they want to learn about an alternative way of living to the one they've been force-fed. People would come up to me and ask, "I want to help; how do I become an activist?" I'd always tell them it's easy: sign a petition; write a letter to the editor; run for town council; start a clothes recycling program at your church; or maybe join a local citizen's group to fight urban sprawl in your community. If you don't feel comfortable doing any of those things, I'd tell them, then eat organic and quit shopping at The Gap. The point is, you don't have to climb the Golden Gate Bridge and hang a banner to be an activist. Just remember the activist's credo: think globally and raise hell locally.

You'll be amazed at how many ways there are to get involved with activist causes when you start to look. The Internet is an activist's dream, a great place to start learning about the issues. One wonderful thing to come out of the whole SOL Tour experience was the website we started, called VoiceYourself.com, so people could keep track of our trip. That website has grown now to become a crossroads for people interested in all the issues related to simple organic living. We talk about the things that are important to us there, connect with fellow activists from across the country and around the world, and provide links so people can connect with non-profit organizations and organic businesses.

I'm proud of what we've been able to do with VoiceYourself.com, but we need more websites like it to provide a forum where people can voice their support for an alternative vision of the world and make connections with other like-minded individuals. In fact, it may be the only way we're ever going to break through, because the corporate media obviously aren't in a big hurry to provide a forum for any idea that might upset the advertisers. After all, the media depends on the culture of consumerism, on the Beast, for its very survival. You can't exactly encourage people to wean themselves off the fossil fuel teat when you're busy trying to sell them a Lincoln Navigator. So we're going to have to build our own direct pathways to get our message out there. The Internet is one way; active protests are another; shopping at your local farmers' market is another.

Most people aren't even aware of it, but we're locked in a struggle right now to determine what the future of this planet is going to look like. Our enemy, the Beast—the corporations that are raping the earth and its people, and the governments and global organizations that support them—has shown that it's a pretty powerful adversary. It has shown it has the power to control commerce, control the media, dominate nations, destroy or alter nature—even to take human life.

I can see how a single individual facing down an enemy like that might feel totally powerless. But you know what? Our side can be pretty powerful too when we get together. We've seen that power on display numerous times in the past. We saw it in the streets of Seattle in 1999 when we shut down the WTO Summit. We saw it back in 1989 when somebody took a hammer and smacked the Berlin Wall and a chunk fell off. Then a few hundred thousand other people took a whack and the whole damn thing came down. That's the power of the people, and there's no power they can create in Washington and no power that money can buy that can equal the power of the people when we move with conviction and in unison.

And that's what we've got to do now. The Beast in all its disguises—the WTO, the International Monetary Fund, the World Bank, the G-8—is trying to steal your right to decide what kind of planet you're going to live on and what kind of planet you're going to leave behind. It's time for all of us to get active and be vigilant in protecting that right. Remember what that great social activist Thomas Jefferson said: "The price of freedom is eternal vigilance." Well, that's what we saw in the streets of Seattle, and that's what we saw before in places like Selma and Kent State: people paying the price for freedom.

For me, activism is a life-long path that we all have a duty to follow. I feel like right now all of us are in a boat in a giant river that's flowing in the wrong direction. Unless we're all paddling as hard as we can against the current, we're going downstream in a hurry. Each one of us, as an individual, can choose to just sit there and do nothing, pretending we're not a part of what's going on. But that attitude is never going to get the boat going in the right direction. No, the only way to fight the current is for all of us to pitch in and do what we can, and every little bit helps. It's like Julia Butterfly Hill says: "Our actions can change the world; our inaction can change the world."

I'm not much for statistics but I've always thought this was an interesting one: When this little activist protest called the American Revolution happened, thirty-five per cent of the population of the colonies was considered loyal to the Crown, meaning they actively supported the British army against the rebels. Another twenty per cent of the population supported the rebellion, meaning they gave food and shelter to the rebel soldiers. The largest percentage, over forty per cent, didn't do shit; they just continued to work their farms and businesses and didn't take sides one way or another. Amazingly, only two per cent were active participants when it came to actually fighting the British army. *Two per cent*—and they succeeded against the most powerful empire in the world at that time. Well, I believe there's a lot more than two per cent of the population today that is feeling disaffected, unrepresented, and disconnected, and we need to get those people moving.

When I was out on the SOL Tour, I had a lot of negative people tell me, "You know Woody, you're only running around preaching to the choir."

"Well, good," I told them, "because if we can get all these choirs singing together with one voice, we're going to make a hell of a noise."

I still feel that way today, and whenever I question my ability to make a difference in the world, I always think back to a quote from the great social anthropologist and humanitarian Margaret Mead: "Never doubt that a small group of thoughtful, committed citizens can change the world. In fact, it's the only thing that ever has."

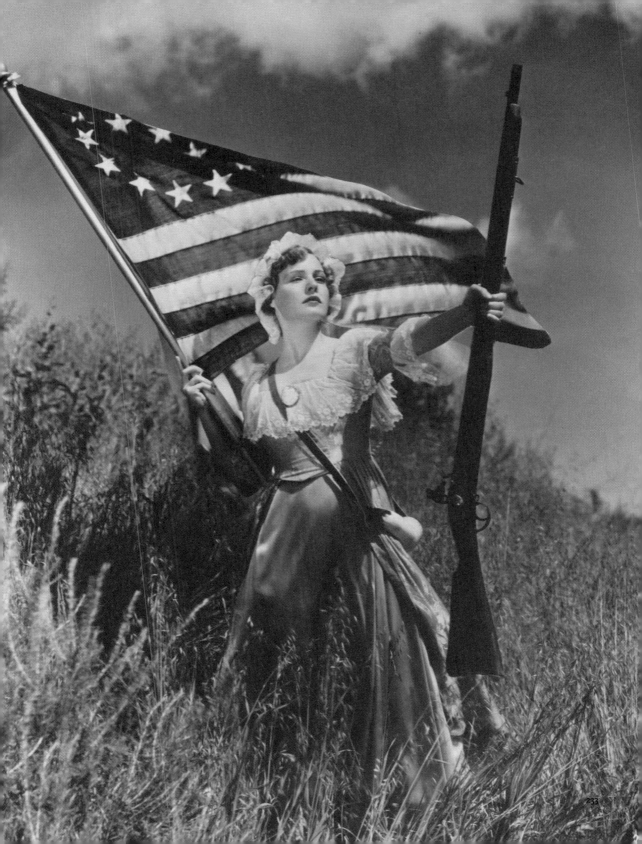

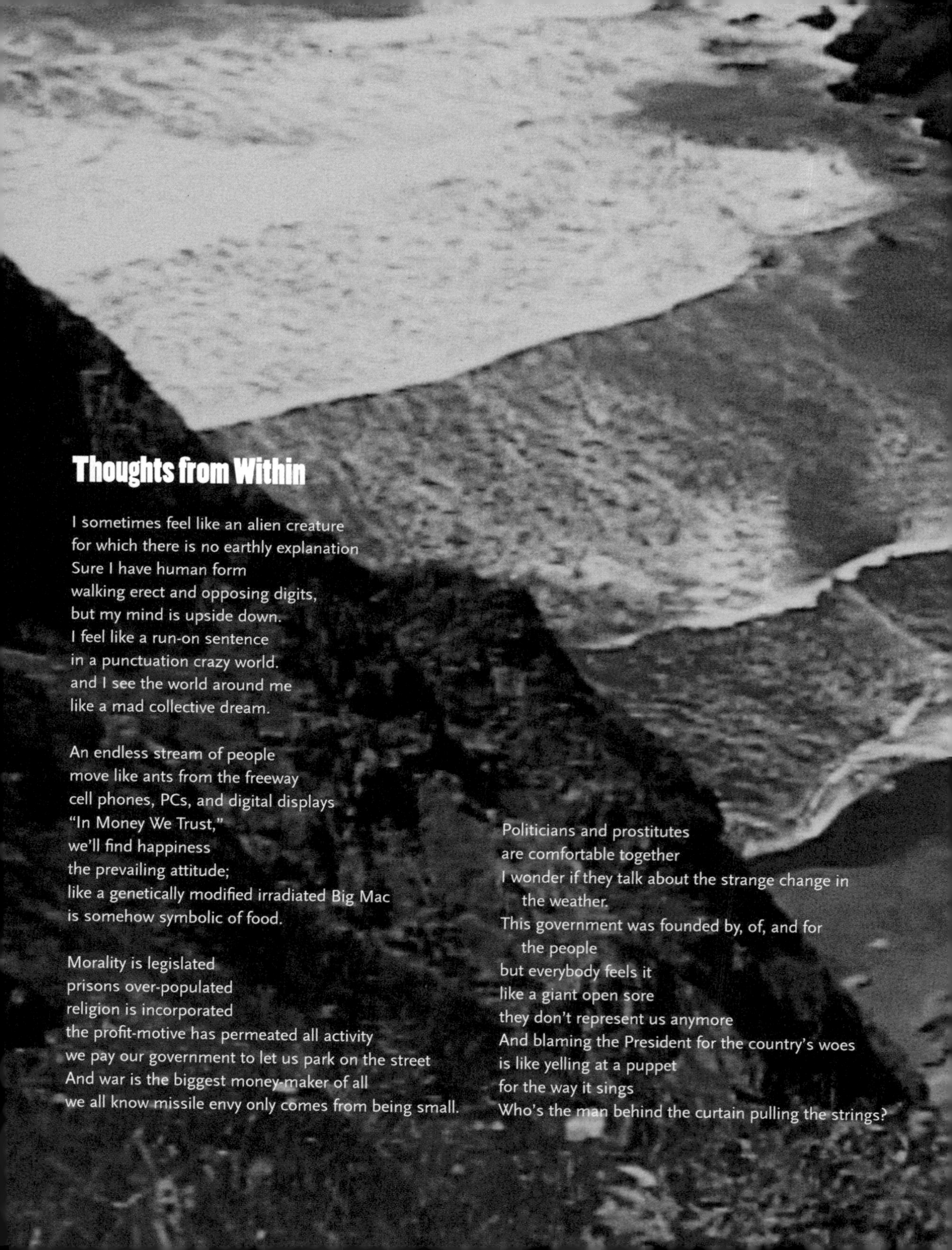

Thoughts from Within

I sometimes feel like an alien creature
for which there is no earthly explanation
Sure I have human form
walking erect and opposing digits,
but my mind is upside down.
I feel like a run-on sentence
in a punctuation crazy world.
and I see the world around me
like a mad collective dream.

An endless stream of people
move like ants from the freeway
cell phones, PCs, and digital displays
"In Money We Trust,"
we'll find happiness
the prevailing attitude;
like a genetically modified irradiated Big Mac
is somehow symbolic of food.

Morality is legislated
prisons over-populated
religion is incorporated
the profit-motive has permeated all activity
we pay our government to let us park on the street
And war is the biggest money-maker of all
we all know missile envy only comes from being small.

Politicians and prostitutes
are comfortable together
I wonder if they talk about the strange change in
   the weather.
This government was founded by, of, and for
   the people
but everybody feels it
like a giant open sore
they don't represent us anymore
And blaming the President for the country's woes
is like yelling at a puppet
for the way it sings
Who's the man behind the curtain pulling the strings?

A billion people sitting watching their TV
in the room that they call living
but as for me
I see living as loving
and since there is no loving room
I sit on the grass under a tree
dreaming of the way things used to be
Pre-Industrial Revolution
which of course is before the rivers and oceans,
    and skies were polluted

before Parkinson's, and mad cows
and all the convoluted cacophony of bad ideas
like skyscrapers, and tree paper, and earth rapers
like Monsanto and Dupont had their way
as they continue to today.

This was Pre-us
back when the buffalo roamed
and the Indian's home
was the forest, and God was nature
and heaven was here and now
Can you imagine clean water, food, and air
living in community with animals and people
    who care?

Do you dare to feel responsible for every dollar
    you lay down
are you going to make the rich man richer
or are you going to stand your ground
You say you want a revolution
a communal evolution
to be a part of the solution
maybe I'll be seeing you around.

—Woody Harrelson

RESOURCES FOR GOING FURTHER

Here are just a few of the many sources of information on how you can "Go Further" in your day-to-day life. Please also see the list of sources for this book for further reading.

Woody Harrelson and Laura Louie's VoiceYourself
http://www.voiceyourself.com
Many of the links below can be clicked on directly from the VoiceYourself site.

The Electric Kool-Aid Acid Test
By Tom Wolfe. New York, NY: Bantam, 1968.

One Flew Over the Cuckoo's Nest
By Ken Kesey. New York, NY: Signet, 1962.

The State of the World..
Various authors. Published annually by the Worldwatch Institute (www.worldwatch.org).

Simple, Sustainable Organic Living:

Alliance for Sustainability
http://allianceforsustainability.net
Aims to bring about planetary sustainability through support of projects that are ecologically sound, economically viable, socially just and humane.

Backhome Magazine
http://www.backhomemagazine.com
A guide to sustainable living focussing on country living skills.

Global Ecovillage Network
http://gen.ecovillage.org
Network encouraging the evolution of sustainable settlements across the world.

Agriculture:

Acres U.S.A.
http://www.acresusa.com/magazines/magazine.htm
Comprehensive guide to sustainable agriculture.

American Farmland Trust
http://www.farmland.org
Since 1980, this trust has helped win permanent protection for over a million acres of American farmland.

Community Alliance with Family Farmers
http://www.caff.org

Ecological Farming Association
http://www.eco-farm.org

Family Farmer
http://www.familyfarmer.org
A national rural community outreach campaign.

Farm to Table
http://www.farmtotable.org
Connects consumers to local farmers to help build an understanding of how our food is grown or raised.

Mad Cowboy
http://www.madcowboy.com
Howard Lyman's web site

Energy:

Alliance to Save Energy
http://www.ase.org
Alliance promoting energy efficiency worldwide.

Apollo Alliance
http://www.apolloalliance.org
Coalition working to free us from our dependency on Middle East oil.

Center for Renewable Energy and Sustainable Technology
http://www.crest.org

Die Off
http://dieoff.org
What could happen when the oil runs out.

Energy & Environmental Building Association
http://www.eeba.org
Promotes development of energy-efficient, environmentally responsible buildings.

Home Power Magazine
http://www.homepower.com
"A journal of homemade power that grew out of our passion for renewable energy."

Real Goods
http://www.realgoods.com
John Schaeffer's company web site.

Hemp:

Global Hemp
http://www.globalhemp.com
Portal to the "hemp community."

Hemp Stores
http://www.hempstores.com
A great database to find what is near you.

Hempology
http://www.hempology.org
Boston Hemp Co-op's digital library and museum on hemp and its history.

Industrial Hemp
http://www.industrialhemp.net
Contains links to organizations, reports and sites all about hemp and issues related to it.

Forests:

American Lands Alliance
http://www.americanlands.org
Offers comprehensive educational and resource materials on major forest issues.

Forest Certification Resource Center
http://www.certifiedwood.org
A guide to products approved by the Forest Stewardship Council, a non-profit that sets standards for sustainable forest management.

Forest Conservation Portal
http://www.forests.org

Future Forests
http://www.futureforests.com
Here you can calculate your carbon dioxide emissions, learn how to reduce them.

Heritage Forest Campaign
http://www.ourforests.org
Working to uphold the protection of America's National Forests.

Natural Resources Defense Council
http://www.nrdc.org
Offers links, news and actions related to forests and forest conservation.

Rainforest Action Network
http://www.ran.org
Works to protect the earth's rainforests and support the rights of their inhabitants.

Activism:

Action! Network Hub
http://actionnetwork.org
Gateway to online activism centers for over 170 environment, health and population advocacy organizations.

Artists Network of Refuse & Resist
http://www.artistsnetwork.org
Creates and promotes art that contributes to a culture of resistance.

Citizen Works
http://www.citizenworks.org
Founded by Ralph Nader in 2001, this non-profit's mandate is to advance justice by strengthening citizen participation in power.

Common Dreams
http://www.commondreams.org
Non-profit citizens' organization using the Internet as a political organizing tool.

Ruckus Society
http://www.ruckus.org
Provides environmental, human rights, and social justice organizers with the tools, training, and support needed to achieve their goals.

Global Warming:

Action Network International
http://www.climatenetwork.org
Global network of NGOs working to limit human-induced climate change.

Early Warning Signs
http://www.climatehotmap.org
Check this map out. It illustrates the local consequences of global warming.

Global Warming International Center
http://www.globalwarming.net
International body that disseminates research information on global warming science and policy.

Air:

Clean Air Council
http://www.cleanair.org
Non-profit organization dedicated to protecting everyone's right to breathe clean air.

Foundation for Clean Air Progress
http://www.cleanairprogress.org
Source for public education and information about improving air quality in America.

Water:

Clean Water Action
http://www.cleanwateraction.org
National citizens' organization working for clean, safe and affordable water.

Global Rivers Environmental Network
http://www.green.org
Educational resources for implementing a school-based water-monitoring program.

Groundwater Foundation
http://www.groundwater.org
Non-profit organization educating and motivating people to care for and about groundwater.

World's Water
http://www.worldwater.org
Provides up-to-date information on a wide range of global freshwater problems and solutions.

Environmental Groups:

Biogems—Saving Endangered Wild Places
http://www.savebiogems.org
BioGems are unspoiled places in the Americas facing imminent destruction from development.

Center for Environmental Citizenship
http://www.envirocitizen.org

Works to increase citizen participation with regard to environmental issues.

Co-op America
http://www.coopamerica.org

Has practical tips for using your consumer and investor power for social change.

Earth Day Network
http://www.earthday.net

Founded by the organizers of the first Earth Day in 1970, this network promotes environmental citizenship and year-round progressive action worldwide.

Earthwatch Institute
http://www.earthwatch.org

Engages people worldwide in scientific field research and education to promote a sustainable environment.

Enviro Link Network
http://www.envirolink.org

Grassroots online community uniting hundreds of organizations and volunteers around the world.

Environmental Defense Fund
http://www.environmentaldefense.org/home.cfm

Dedicated to protecting the environmental rights of all people, including future generations.

Friends of the Earth
http://www.foe.co.uk

One of the largest international networks of environmental groups, represented in over 70 countries.

Greenpeace
http://www.greenpeaceusa.org

This famous organization uses non-violent direct action and creative communication to expose global environmental problems.

Nature Conservancy
http://nature.org

Works to preserve the plants, animals and natural communities that represent the diversity of life on earth.

Oceana
http://www.oceana.org

Campaigns to protect and restore the world's oceans.

Redefining Progress
http://www.rprogress.org
Calculate your community's "Ecological Footprint."

Save Our Environment
http://www.saveourenvironment.org/action
Collaborative effort of the nation's most influential environmental advocacy organizations harnessing the power of the Internet to increase public awareness and activism on today's most important environmental issues.

Sprawl Watch
http://www.sprawlwatch.org
Clearinghouse on sustainable growth.

Surfrider
http://www.surfrider.org
Surfers share their first-hand knowledge of the state of our oceans and beaches.

Union of Concerned Scientists
http://www.ucsusa.org
Alliance of citizens and scientists augmenting rigorous scientific analysis with innovative thinking and committed citizen advocacy to build a cleaner, healthier environment and a safer world.

World Wildlife Fund
http://www.worldwildlife.org
Leads international efforts to protect endangered species and their habitats.

Youth for Environmental Sanity (YES)
http://www.yesworld.org
Non-profit organization that empowers young change-makers to join forces for a sustainable way of life for all.

Alternative Media:

Cascadia Media Collective
http://www.cascadiamedia.org
Guerrilla journalists producing multimedia projects on social injustice and environmental destruction.

Environmental Media Association
http://www.ema-online.org
Helps environmental groups convey their message in the most effective way possible.

MediaWatch
http://www.mediawatch.org
Collects a number of alternative media sites on one homepage.

Undercurrents
http://www.undercurrents.org
For news you don't get on the news.

Video Activism
http://www.videoactivism.org
Informal association of activists and artists using video to support social, economic and environmental justice campaigns.

Web Active
http://www.webactive.com
A collection of alternative radio stations and information.

Witness
http://www.witness.org
A human rights online video program. Co-founded by Peter Gabriel.

Yoga:

Yoga Basics
http://www.yogabasics.com/
Commercial site with introductory articles on yoga.

The Yoga Site
http://www.yogasite.com/articles.htm
Commercial site primarily selling yoga accessories but also has interesting articles on the uses of yoga.

Yoga Journal
http://www.yogajournal.com/
Website for the bi-monthly print magazine.

Raw Food:

Living Cuisine: The Art and Spirit of Raw Foods
By Renée Loux Underkoffler. Toronto, ON: Penguin Books (Avery Health Guides), 2004.

SOURCES

American Cancer Society. "Who gets cancer?" <http://www.cancer.org/docroot/CRI/content/CRI_2_4_1x_Who_gets_cancer.asp?sitearea=>.

Aronson, E. & O'Leary, M. (1983). "The relative effectiveness of models and prompts on energy conservation: a field experiment in a shower room." *Journal of Environmental Systems*, 12, 219–224.

Drug Sense. "War on Drugs Clock". <http://www.drugsense.org/wodclock.htm> (accessed November 2004).

Friends of the Earth. "Chronology of the Exposé of Genetically Engineered StarLink™ Corn Not Approved for Human Consumption." <http://www.foe.org/camps/comm/safefood/gefood/foodaid/news.html>

Green, Ché. "Got rGBH?" *Independent Weekly*, August 7, 2002. <http://www.indyweek.com/durham/2002-08-07/cover.html>.

Groth, Edward, et al. *Do You Know What You're Eating? An analysis of U.S. government data on pesticide residues in food.* Washington, DC: Consumers Union, 1999.<http://www.consumersunion.org/food/do_you_know2.htm>.

Gulland, Anne. "Air pollution responsible for 600,000 premature deaths worldwide," BMJ Dec. 14, 2002 <http://bmj.bmjjournals.com/cgi/content/full/325/7377/1380/c>.

Jolly, Richard, et al. *Human Development Report 1998* (New York: United Nations Development Programme, 1998). PDF available at <http://hdr.undp.org/reports/global/1998/en/>.

Lee, Maxwell. "History of Vegetarianism." The Vegetarian Society of the United Kingdom web site <http://www.vegsoc.org/info/developm.html> (accessed August 2004).

Living-Foods.com. "The Living and Raw Foods F.A.Q. (Frequently Asked Questions)." <http://www.living-foods.com/faq.html> (accessed August 2004).

Magazine Paper Project (Co-op America). "How Many Trees Logged for Your Magazine?" August 28, 2002. <http://www.ecopaperaction.org/news1.html>.

Mokdad, Ali H., PhD, James S. Marks, MD, MPH, Donna F. Stroup, PhD, MSc, Julie L. Gerberding, MD, MPH, "Actual Causes of Death in the United States, 2000," *Journal of the American Medical Association,* March 10, 2004, Vol. 291, No. 10, p. 1242. Available as a PDF at <http://www.drugwarfacts.org/causes.htm>.

National Center For Chronic Disease Prevention and Health Promotion. "Cigarette Smoking–Related Mortality." June 2001. <http://www.cdc.gov/tobacco/research_data/health_consequences/mortali.htm>

National Highway Traffic Safety Administration (NHTSA). "States' Progress Drops Drunk Driving Deaths To Lowest Level Since 1999." August 25, 2004 <http://www.nhtsa.dot.gov/hot/press-display.cfm?year=2004&filename=pr38-04.html>

Organic Consumers Association. "Monsanto Brings Small Family Dairy to Court." <http://www.organic-consumers.org/monlink.html#farmers> (accessed November 2004).

Pierce, Karn. "No Bag, Thanks." Australian broadcasting corporation Science Online. <http://www.abc.net.au/science/features/bags/default.htm>. Accessed August 2004.

Ransom, David. *The No-Nonsense Guide to Fair Trade.* Second edition. Toronto: New Internationalist Publications Ltd., 2002.

Roach, John. "Are Plastic Grocery Bags Sacking the Environment?" *National Geographic News,* September 2, 2003. <http://news.nationalgeographic.com/news/2003/09/0902_030902_plasticbags.html>.

Sierra Club, "Pulp Facts: The environmental impact of wood and paper consumption," <http://www.sierraclub.org/sustainable_consumption/factsheets/forestproducts_factsheet.asp>.

Steger, Manfred B. *Globalization: A Very Short Introduction.* Oxford: Oxford University Press, 2003.

Stepaniak, Joanne. *The Ultimate Uncheese Cookbook.* Summertown, TN: Book Publishing Company, 2003.

Sustainable Table. "The Issues: Organic." <http://www.sustainabletable.org/issues/organic/> (accessed August 2004).

Szoboszlay, Akos. "Conflict of Transportation Competitors," Modern Transit Society web site. January 1999. <http://www.trainweb.org/mts/ctc/index.html>.

Union of Concerned Scientists. "Global warming is real and underway." July 11, 2003. <http://www.ucsusa.org/global_environment/global_warming/index.cfm>.

USDA Agricultural Marketing Service. "The National Organic Program: Labeling and Marketing Information," USDA, October 2002. <http://www.ams.usda.gov/nop/FactSheets/LabelingE.html>.

Vegan Society, The. "History." <http://www.vegansociety.com/html/about_us/history/>.

Williams, Jessica. *50 Facts That Should Change the World.* Cambridge, UK: Icon Books Ltd., 2004.

Williams, Tad. *The Corruption of American Agriculture* (Washington, DC: Americans for Democratic Action Education Fund, n.d.; <www.adaction.org/TadFinal.pdf>.

Woodwise (Co-op America). "Woodwise Consumer Guide." <http://www.woodwise.org/guide/guidehome.html>.

PHOTO CREDITS

This page constitutes an extension of the copyright page. All images used in this book, including the covers, are from the production of the film *Go Further* by Sphinx Productions, except as noted below. All effort has been made to contact copyright holders.

Pages 2–7, 39, 40, 42, 46, 48, 54, 58–59, 67, 72–73 (book background), 88–90, 94, 99, 100 (paper background), 107–111, 115, 128, 141, 142, 148, 169, 171, 174, 176–77, 178, 182–83: ©Photospin.

Pages 164, 172–73, 180–81: ©Colin Finlay, Photospin.

Pages 28–29: Courtesy of Jim Williamson.

Page 43: Corporate American flag image courtesy of AdBusters. Flag may be purchased through www.unbrandamerica.org.

Pages 70–71: IH070629 Harvesting Organic Carrots © Paul A. Souders/Corbis/Magma

Page 131: 0000337265-001 Oprah Winfrey © R.Mulherin/Corbis Sygma/Magma

Pages 152–53: BE023015 "Washington Crossing the Delaware" by Emanuel Gottlieb Leutze © Bettmann/Corbis/Magma

Pages 156–57: CSM106592 Field of Hemp Plants ©Jim Craigmyle/Corbis/Magma

Pages 160–61: CSM106585 Hemp Growing in Field ©Jim Craigmyle/Corbis/Magma

Page 187: AAJC001477 George W. Bush ©Brooks Kraft/Corbis/Magma

Pages 196–97: HU028120 Women Processing Hemp to Make Rigging for the Royal Navy, ca. 1956 ©Hulton-Deutsch Collection/Corbis/Magma

Pages 208–209 0000212327-006 Greenpeace Ship Moored off Tahiti ©Jacques Langevin/Corbis Sygma/Magma

Page 210: 0000307149-012 Bill Clinton On Official Visit in Ukraine ©McNamee Wally/Corbis Sygma/Magma

Pages 214–15: AAFG001461 Police Controlling Demonstrators Against WTO ©David Butow/Corbis Saba/Magma

Pages 216–17: AAFR001311 Police in Riot Gear During WTO Protests ©Christopher J. Morris/Corbis/Magma

Page 222: 0000360392-004 Demonstration Against WTO Conference ©Touhig Sion/Corbis Sygma/Magma

Pages 224–25: 0000320552-002 Greenpeace Protest in the Bering Sea ©R. Visser/Greenpeace/Corbis Sygma/Magma

Pages 226–27: 0000341715-005 Julia Butterfly Hill © Corbis Sygma/Magma

Page 233: JS1563069 Actress Madge Evans ©John Springer Collection/Corbis/Magma

Page 131: Courtesy of Howard Lyman, www.madcowboy.com.

Pages 149–51, 154, 158: From the film *Grass* ©Sphinx Productions, courtesy of Warwick Publishing.

Page 184: Courtesy of John Schaeffer, www.realgoods.com.

Pages 202, 204, 207: ©Malcolm MacKinnon.

Page 211: Courtesy of Twilly Cannon.

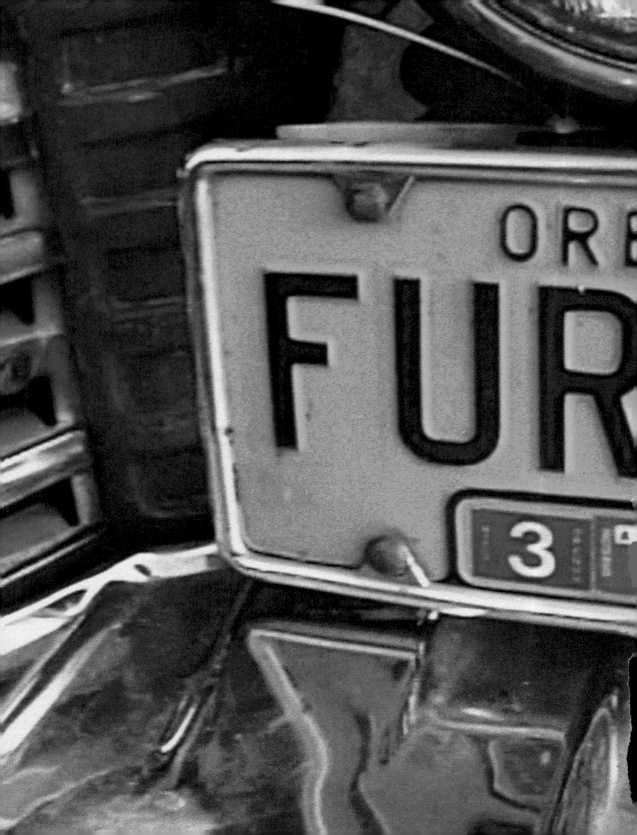

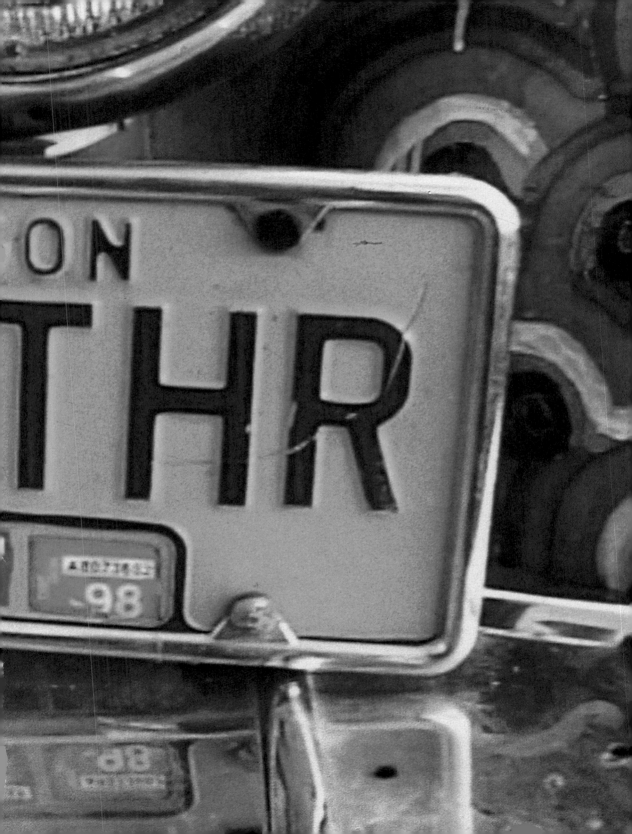

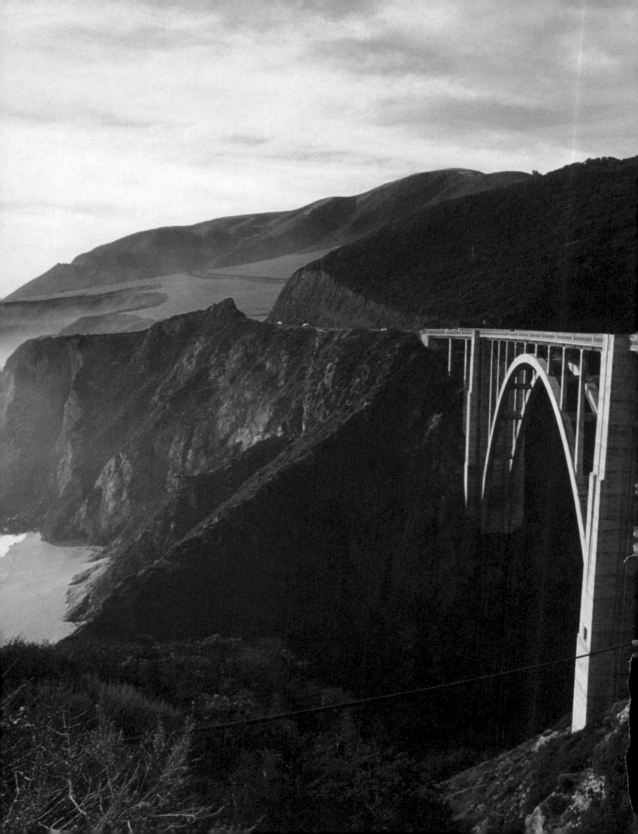